HEALTHY EATING
GLUTEN-FREE

Tasty recipes for coeliac disease

Authors: Trudel Marquardt, Britta-Marei Lanzenberger

Photography: Michael Brauner

NEW
HOLLAND

CONTENTS

A GLUTEN-FREE DIET

Enjoying your meals –
   in spite of coeliac disease   5

Coeliac disease –
   illness through grain   6

Questions and answers –
   identifying symptoms and reacting   8

In practice –
   living with coeliac disease   10

The intestine –
   a weakened immune system   12

Questions and answers –
   important facts for everyday routines   14

The diagnosis   16

My child has coeliac disease   17

Questions and answers –
   general questions   18

Initial steps after diagnosis   20

Questions and Answers –
   gluten-free baking   22

RECIPES

Soups and Sauces

Vegetable soup with polenta gnocchi,
   Cream of mushroom soup   26

Tasty tomato sauce, Béchamel sauce   28

Spicy barbecue sauce,
   Creamy curry sauce   29

Pasta Dishes

Gnocchi with parmesan   30

Cheesy polenta bake   32

Penne with zucchini sauce,
   Spaghetti carbonara   34

Lasagne   36

Meaty pasta parcels   38

Main Courses

Pickled beef roast with bread dumplings   40

Pancake wraps with meat filling   42

Burritos with chicken filling   44

Zucchini tortilla   46

Savoury Baking

Basic recipe pizza dough, Focaccia   48

Colourful family pizza   50

Polenta pizza   52

Basic recipe yeast dough,
   French onion tart   54

Basic recipe cream cheese and oil pastry,
   Basic recipe cream cheese puff pastry   56

Meat parcels   58

Leek quiche   60

Cheese bites   62

Desserts

French apple crumble,
  Red jelly with custard 64

Light orange mousse,
  Scandinavian buttermilk cream 66

Belgian waffles,
  German cream cheese potato cakes 68

Rice and cream cheese gratin with apples,
  Sweet millet gratin 70

Raspberry tiramisu,
  Basic recipe sponge cake 72

Cakes and Gateaux

Raspberry cream cake,
  Cheesecake without base 74

Fruity walnut muffins,
  Chocolate and almond muffins 76

Coconut & orange muffins, Almond slice 78

Espresso cake, Buckwheat cake 80

French cherry gâteau,
  Lemon cake 82

Swiss carrot cake 84

Almond cake 86

Basic recipe shortcrust pastry,
  Rhubarb cake with custard topping 88

Gooseberry cake,
  Apple cake with cinnamon frosting 90

Linzer torte 92

Christmas Baking

Butter biscuits 94

Fancy pistachio fingers, Lemon hearts 96

Coconut & marzipan macaroons,
  Hazelnut macaroons 98

Almond crescents, Chocolate slices 100

Mini meringues, Walnut cookies 102

Breads and Rolls

Weekend bread rolls 104

Wholemeal bread rolls or wholemeal
  bread, Yeast-free bread rolls 106

White bread rolls or white bread 108

Potato bread, Rice bread 110

Multigrain yoghurt bread 112

Amaranth bread with linseed, Walnut bread 114

Bread without using a bread mix 116

My favourite bread 118

LOOK IT UP

Glossary 120

Weekly menu plan 124

Food chart 126

Recipes index – by chapter 129

Index 130

Imprint 132

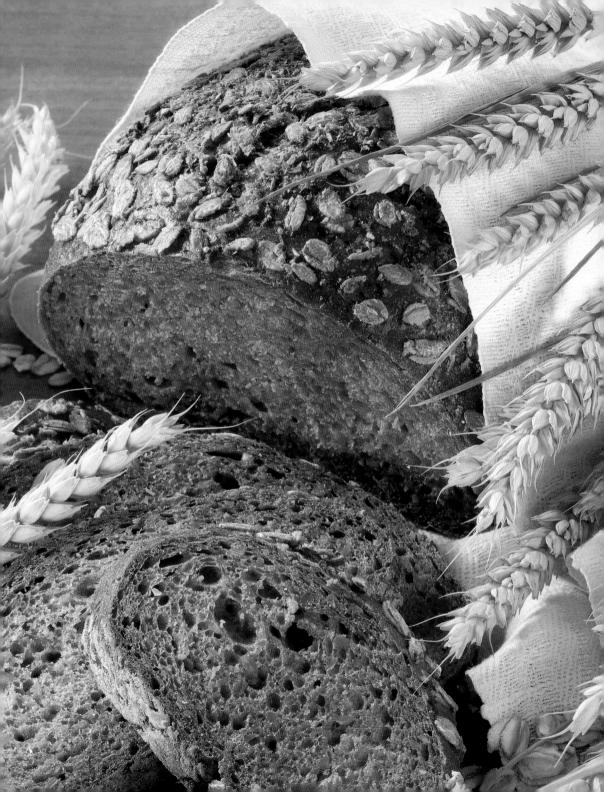

ENJOYING YOUR MEALS IN SPITE OF
COELIAC DISEASE
THANKS TO THE RIGHT RECIPE CHOICE

The hidden risks of eating grains – while a healthy staple food for most people, it can be life-threatening for coeliac sufferers.

Wheat, barley, rye and spelt are considered healthy foods, but some people react with an intolerance to these grain varieties. This is due to the grain protein, known as gluten, which can cause life-threatening inflammations if it reaches the small intestine in those who are affected. Coeliac disease is particularly common among children, but adults can also develop a sudden intolerance to the gluten in grains. The exact reasons for this remain unclear. The only treatment is a life-long diet. This guide will help you answer any questions you may have about gluten-free food, offering tips and tricks for successful, tasty, gluten-free cooking and baking.

COELIAC DISEASE
ILLNESS THROUGH GRAIN

COELIAC DISEASE OR SPRUE?

In 1888, an English doctor described the illness of one of his young patients as a "coeliac affection", derived from the Greek word "koilia" for stomach. The English word "coeliac" is also based on this word.

Without knowing the cause of the disease, people tried out various diets, such as a banana diet and a fruit and vegetable diet. It was not until 1950 that a team of Dutch paediatricians found the disease to be triggered by the grain protein, gluten. The team also discovered that the disease generally known as "sprue" in adults had the same causes. In the case of sprue, a distinction is also made between "coeliac sprue" and "tropical sprue", as these are two medically different disorders.

This resulted in there being two names for what is actually the same disease: coeliac disease in children and sprue in adults, although this distinction is normally only made in the United States and not in England or Australia, where it is known only as "coeliac disease".

WHAT IS GLUTEN?

Grains contain up to 15 percent protein. In the most widely used cereals – wheat, rye, barley and oats – this protein is almost entirely gluten, which, as a binding protein, keeps the dough elastic during processing. Flours containing gluten are therefore particularly well suited, and thus the number one choice for baking breads, cakes and all kinds of pastries.

Apart from grains and grain products, gluten is also found in a large number of ready-made meals. Thanks to its excellent properties as a binder, emulsifier and stabiliser for water, gluten is commonly used for a variety of purposes in the food industry.

The gluten in these grain varieties has different names:

GRAIN	GLUTEN
wheat	gliadin
rye	secalin
barley	hordein
oats	avenin

WHAT IS COELIAC DISEASE?

People suffering from coeliac disease react with an intolerance to the presence of the grain protein, gluten. If the gluten gets into their small intestine, it activates the immune system, causing the intestinal mucosa to inflame. This damages the surface of the mucous membrane, making it impossible for it to be regenerated in the long run. Food can thus no longer be utilised sufficiently and to its full extent, resulting in an energy and nutrient deficiency. The immune system is constantly active, and the body must continuously fight against an inflammation.

WHO CAN CONTRACT COELIAC DISEASE?

Although many people may be genetically pre-disposed to contracting coeliac disease, genes are not the sole cause for the disease to occur. Studies show that 70 percent of identical twins suffer from it, with this figure being 30 percent in genetically similar siblings, and 10 percent in immediate relatives.

If genes were wholly and solely responsible, coeliac disease would be more prevalent in the affected families. This means that, although pre-disposition is hereditary, other factors can also play a role.

The disease can appear at any age, and is most frequently diagnosed in infants who react to their first gluten-containing food with the typical symptoms. In adults, it is most common between the ages of 30 and 40. However, as many years can pass between the disease developing and it being diagnosed, the actual point at which it starts is often unclear.

HOW COMMON IS COELIAC DISEASE?

Figures on the disease's prevalence fluctuate significantly, but it affects approximately 1 in 100 Australians. However, as many symptoms are not identified as being those of coeliac disease, 75 percent of cases currently remain undiagnosed, meaning 157,000 Australians have the disease without realising it. Conversely, the disease is virtually unheard of in China, Japan and Africa, which is probably due to both genetic pre-disposition and other eating habits involving fewer cereals and more rice. Women are somewhat more likely to contract coeliac disease than men, with a ratio of 2 or 3 to 1. Prevalence in babies has decreased since

the 1970s, as they are now being breastfed for longer and introduced to gluten-containing foods at a later stage. It is uncertain whether this reduces the risk of contracting the disease altogether or just postpones its appearance.

WHICH FACTORS INFLUENCE CONTRACTION OF THE DISEASE?

As the causes of coeliac disease are still largely unclear, nobody knows which factors influence actual contraction of the disease. There has been a noticeable general increase in the prevalence of coeliac disease over the last few decades – with very vague symptoms in some cases. What is debatable is whether better diagnostic facilities also play a role in this rise of cases. Environmental factors, incorrect eating habits, infections or stress are all suspected of causing the increased prevalence.

CONSEQUENCES OF UNDETECTED COELIAC DISEASE

> iron deficiency (anaemia)
> night blindness (nyctalopia)
> tendency to bleed (haemophilia)
> sore bones/Osteoporosis
> rickets
> oedema (fluid retention)
> muscle cramps
> menstrual problems
> infertility, premature births, miscarriages
> depression
> susceptibility to infection
> poor wound healing
> bowel cancer

IDENTIFYING
SYMPTOMS AND REACTING

1. ARE PEOPLE GENETICALLY PREDISPOSED TO COELIAC DISEASE, AND IS IT HEREDITARY?

The risk of contracting coeliac disease does depend on genes. Studies have shown that 70 percent of identical twins contract it. However, a genetic predisposition does not necessarily mean that the disease will actually appear. Additional triggers are still unclear.

2. IS COELIAC DISEASE AN ALLERGY OR AN INTOLERANCE?

Coeliac disease is a special type of food intolerance. The immune system is activated by the intestine's reaction to the presence of gluten. The intestinal mucosa then becomes inflamed, the intestinal villi are flattened, and new villi are no longer able to form properly, meaning food components cannot be sufficiently taken up by the body.

3. IS THERE A CURE FOR COELIAC DISEASE?

All symptoms of coeliac disease can dissipate if a gluten-free diet is strictly adhered to. As long as incorrect eating habits are avoided, there is no heightened risk of secondary diseases. However, gluten intolerances are unfortunately – in most cases – a life-long affliction. There are currently no medications to relieve or cure it.

4. HOW LONG DOES IT TAKE TO RECOVER?

That depends on how long the coeliac disease has been present and how badly the intestinal villi have been damaged. However, the intestine can recover relatively quickly if it is not aggravated by more gluten. There is normally a noticeable improvement after around three weeks, although this can also be longer depending on the individual.

5. WHAT ARE THE POSSIBLE CONSEQUENCES IF COELIAC DISEASE GOES UNDETECTED FOR A LONG TIME?

If coeliac disease has gone undetected for some time, there is an increased risk of deficiency symptoms due to the intestinal damage. A vitamin and mineral deficiency can have numerous health consequences, which can cause permanent damage in children. The risk of bowel cancer is also higher.

6. CAN THE BODY COMPLETELY REGENERATE ITSELF?

The body has fantastic self-healing powers, enabling it to counteract almost all damage. If a gluten-free diet is strictly maintained, the intestine can recover within about one year. It is very important, however, to help the body with its healing process, and to lead a lifestyle which is as holistically healthy as possible.

7. HOW HIGH IS THE RISK OF DEVELOPING A MALIGNANT TUMOUR?

People with coeliac disease are at no higher risk of cancer if a gluten-free diet is strictly maintained. Careful selection of food can actually create an opportunity to have a particularly healthy diet, which is why incorrect eating habits must be avoided, and gluten-free diets should always be considered an active form of cancer prevention.

8. CAN I EAT NORMALLY AGAIN IF I HAVEN'T HAD ANY SYMPTOMS FOR YEARS?

Do not, under any circumstances, take it upon yourself to test whether you can tolerate gluten-containing foods again after a long period of no symptoms. You have to assume that the lack of symptoms is solely the result of your gluten-free diet. Trying out gluten-containing foods always involves a very high risk of relapse, and increases the risk of bowel cancer.

9. ARE A FEW UNHEALTHY EATING HABITS REALLY SO BAD?

One single unhealthy or incorrect eating habit can trigger an immediate outbreak. However, it is also possible that no noticeable symptoms will appear. In any case, such eating habits mean more damage to the intestine and a strain on the immune system, thereby increasing the risk of developing a malignant tumour.

IN PRACTICE
LIVING WITH COELIAC DISEASE

IS THERE A CURE FOR COELIAC DISEASE?

Generally, no. Although some cases of apparent "cure" have been recorded, these may also have been due to incorrect diagnoses having been made previously. If diagnosed reliably, it must be assumed that the intolerance will persist for life. All reports and miracle cures promising the contrary should therefore be critically questioned.

On rare occasions, cures have been observed in infants diagnosed with the disease before their first birthday, but this possibility must be confirmed by detailed, regular examinations, as the risk of damage would be too high.

Although a gluten-free diet is not a cure for coeliac disease, it does prevent any symptoms from appearing.

THE ONLY TREATMENT: A GLUTEN-FREE DIET

The only possible treatment of coeliac disease is a totally gluten-free diet. So far, no type of successful medication is available. However, in acute cases, there are various options for soothing the aggravated intestinal mucosa and helping the intestine's healing process. A holistic medical practitioner or alternative practitioner can assist you with this.

SYMPTOMS OF COELIAC DISEASE

> digestion problems
> diarrhoea
> greasy, bulky stools
> flatulence
> nausea
> tiredness
> abnormal fatigue
> general malaise
> depression
> lack of appetite
> food binges
> weight loss
> in young people:
  – delayed puberty
  – arrested growth

As high levels of stress are also suspected of playing a part in coeliac disease, try to avoid stressful situations, or find a way of managing your stress, for example with the help of meditation or yoga. There are now also special relaxation methods available for the gastro-intestinal region. Plenty of physical exercise, fresh air and breathing exercises can further complement the treatment and help you to feel better.

Damaged intestinal mucosa can be easily penetrated by all kinds of harmful substances, which is why you should always give preference to organic foods and try to avoid all the so-called stimulants, such as tobacco, alcohol and sweets.

CAN COELIAC DISEASE BE PREVENTED?

As the causes of coeliac disease are unclear, there are no specific prevention recommendations available for adults, although it is always advisable to maintain as healthy a lifestyle and diet as possible.

Infants whose parents have coeliac disease should be breastfed for at least six months where possible. This allows sound development of intestinal flora and the immune system. Adding solids to their diet as late as possible prevents early contact with the potentially problematic grain protein. It is also a good idea to try each type of food separately and to keep a close eye on a possible reaction. It is particularly important to pay attention to possible symptoms when first introducing the child to food containing grains. If the infant reacts with vomiting, flatulence and diarrhoea, they should not be fed the mash again. However, parents with coeliac disease should not, under any circumstances, deprive their child of glutenous foods without the disease having been reliably diagnosed. Grains should not be removed from an adult's or child's diet purely based on suspicion. If the relevant symptoms then do appear, it is important to ascertain the exact causes of these.

Children in families affected by coeliac disease can undergo a blood test as a precaution. If the result is negative and no symptoms are apparent, it is very likely the child does not have coeliac disease. If the result is positive, a biopsy should be taken to erase all doubt.

DIETS AS PROTECTION AGAINST CANCER

Sufferers of coeliac disease are at no greater health risk than anyone else – provided they maintain a gluten-free diet. Due to the limited range of foods available, it is important to ensure a well-balanced

SYMPTOMS IN INFANTS

> growth disturbances
> general failure to thrive
> flatulence
> bloated, distended stomach
> diarrhoea
> greasy, bulky stools
> pallor
> vomiting
> personality changes
> weepiness
> disinterest
> social withdrawal
> lack of appetite
> muscular weakness (amyosthenia)

diet. This creates an opportunity to eat particularly healthy foods which prevent general health risks. The risk of the aforementioned side-effects and diseases only increases if the diet is not maintained. Even the smallest quantities of gluten can damage the intestine, increasing the risk of bowel cancer by tenfold.

WHAT SHOULD I DO IF I EAT THE WRONG THING?

In general, you should always be extremely vigilant to ensure you don't eat the "wrong things". There is no such thing as "kind of" gluten-free. Although noticeable symptoms will not necessarily appear if gluten-containing foods are consumed by mistake, this will still activate the immune system and damage the intestinal mucosa.

Any incorrect dietary habit can thus pose a serious risk to your health. If you experience stomach pain and diarrhoea, the cause should be ascertained in order to prevent the same mistake being made again.

THE INTESTINE
A WEAKENED IMMUNE SYSTEM

THE SMALL INTESTINE

While our outer skin measures 2 sq m (21.5 sq ft), the "inner skin" of our intestinal tract is between 500 and 700 sq m (5,380 and 7,532 sq ft). The small intestine of a person with coeliac disease covers 120 sq m (1,290 sq ft) of this, spanning a length of between 3 and 5 m (10 and 16.5 ft). This is only possible thanks to a highly complex structure – folded into an extremely narrow space, the mucous surface area of about 600 circular folds (plicae circulares) is enlarged to 1 sq m (11 sq ft). One cubic millimetre of this area contains up to 40 intestinal villi, which, with a height of 1 mm and a diameter of 0.1 mm, expand the surface area to 5–6 sq m (54–64.5 sq ft). One cubic millimetre of each intestinal villus in turn, comprises 200 million microvilli, which, if laid out, would be as big as a football field.

This vast surface area with its complex structure is necessary for the proper absorption of food. Each villus is made up of microscopic arteries and veins, and is criss-crossed by a network of blood capillaries and lymph vessels. It is this network which enables nutrients to be absorbed and passed into the blood. When someone has coeliac disease, constant inflammation destroys these villi, making it impossible for new villi to grow back. The medical term for this is "villous atrophy" – a lively "hilly landscape" is replaced by a smooth surface which, with its much smaller surface area, cannot sufficiently absorb the nutritional components.

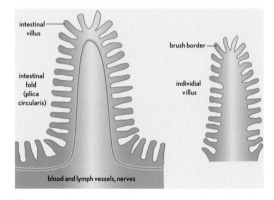

The intestinal mucosa unfolds into creases, villi and brush borders, enlarging the total intestinal surface area by a factor of 200.

THE INTESTINAL FLORA

The stomach contents must first be broken down into their tiniest individual chemical components. Billions of healthy bacteria live in our intestine in order to complete this task for us. We call this ecosystem the "intestinal flora". A healthy intestinal flora composition depends on both our lifestyle and the type of food we customarily eat. Our overall health is directly influenced by our intestinal flora. In coeliac sufferers, the intestinal flora's composition is affected and no longer at the optimum level necessary to maintain good health and symptom-free living.

THE INTESTINE, OUR BIGGEST IMMUNE SYSTEM

Both the outer and inner skin act as our body's threshold to the outside world. At this threshold, it is important to ensure that vital substances can enter the body, while keeping the harmful ones out. By eating, we expose our intestinal tract to dangerous substances several times a day. Along with healthy nutrients, there are also a number of unhealthy components present, such as bacteria or fungi, which the body must detect, reject and eliminate.

It is for this reason that the largest section of the immune system (about 70–80 percent) is situated within the intestine, where it is able to ensure as smooth a process as possible, making it responsible for maintaining the overall health of the body.

THE IMMUNE SYSTEM

Special cells in the body are programmed to detect and reject foreign substances. Upon initial contact, they are programmed to detect these substances. If

WHAT HARMS THE INTESTINE

> denatured foods
> fast food
> hard-to-digest foods
> sugar
> too much fat
> not enough fluid
> alcohol
> nicotine
> medications
> stress and emotional distress
> shallow breathing
> tight clothing (pants, skirts)
> not enough exercise
> eating too quickly

WHAT HELPS THE INTESTINE

> fresh food
> careful food preparation
> dietary fibres
> easily digestible foods
> plenty of fluid (still water)
> herbal teas
> exercise
> relaxation
> breathing exercises
> fresh air
> proper chewing
> control of symbiosis
> homeopathy
> positive attitude towards life

the body comes into contact with them a second time, the cells detect the substances again, latch onto them immediately and thus ensure that they cannot cause any damage. This is known as the "lock and key principle".

This vital process can also apply to substances which are not actually harmful. The immune system reacts in a hypersensitive manner and wrongly treats normal and everyday substances as if they were hostile invaders. Basically, it goes crazy – resulting in an allergy.

In the case of coeliac disease, the grain component, gluten, is incorrectly identified by the body as a harmful substance. The immune system is alerted by the antigen and produces defence cells: the so-called "antibodies". It is these antibodies that cause the intestinal mucosa to inflame, damaging the body's own tissue – and this is the reason why coeliac disease is classed as an "autoimmune disease". The exact processes that occur within the body during an autoimmune response, causing it to attack its own cells, are not yet fully understood but researchers are trying to address these issues.

IMPORTANT FACTS
FOR EVERYDAY ROUTINES

1. DO SYMPTOMS APPEAR IMMEDIATELY IF THE WRONG FOODS ARE EATEN?

If foods containing gluten are consumed, this does not necessarily mean you will directly experience symptoms. Intestinal damage does not become immediately apparent through symptoms. Coeliac disease can break out later due to stress or other adverse factors. As the disease is more advanced at this stage it requires particularly strict discipline.

2. WHAT ELSE CAN HELP, APART FROM A GLUTEN-FREE DIET?

Apart from eating strictly gluten-free foods, you should also be sure to maintain a healthy, balanced diet in general. All foods which do not unnecessarily affect or aggravate the intestine are recommended. Anything which is spicy, acidic or hard to digest should best be replaced with mild foods rich in dietary fibre.

3. DOES A GLUTEN-FREE DIET CAUSE NUTRIENT DEFICIENCIES?

Although a gluten-free diet requires you to eliminate some foods from your eating habits, you don't need to worry about this causing a nutrient deficiency. A balanced diet with fresh ingredients prevents any such deficiency. Where possible, buy seasonal organic produce and prepare this in a careful, health-conscious manner.

4. IS IT A GOOD IDEA TO TAKE DIETARY SUPPLEMENTS?

It can be a good idea for coeliac sufferers to take dietary supplements. They can provide balance if there is a nutrient deficiency and also help the intestinal mucosa to heal. But supplements should never be taken haphazardly. Discuss any necessary supplement with your doctor or alternative practitioner, and give preference to high-quality natural products without glutenous additives.

5. HOW CAN I HELP THE HEALING PROCESS?

Anything which soothes the intestine will help it to heal. This includes healing clay, psyllium husks, linseed and aloe vera. Basic (alkaline) substances help to negate hyperacidity. Ask your doctor or alternative practitioner about promoting symbiosis among intestinal flora. Recovery is aided by general relaxation, exercising in fresh air and minimising the stress you are exposed to.

6. CAN I GO ON HOLIDAY IF I HAVE COELIAC DISEASE?

Plan your holiday carefully to ensure you can relax and not have to run the risk of a relapse while you are away. Read up on local shopping options beforehand, and take some gluten-free food and ingredients with you if necessary. Look out for accommodation offering gluten-free cuisine or where you can cook for yourself. The "Gluten Free Travel Guide" published by the Coeliac Society of Victoria is very helpful.

7. WHAT DO I DO IF I AM INVITED TO A MEAL?

The best thing is to inform your host in advance of your needs and ask whether there will be any gluten-free dishes. They may be able to cater to your dietary requirements, or else you may be able to bring your own gluten-free meal along. If invited to coffee, every host will love it if you bring a cake you baked yourself.

8. DINING OUT WITH COELIAC DISEASE

At restaurants, you must select gluten-free dishes from the menu wherever possible, and ask the chef about ingredients and preparation methods. Sometimes it is helpful to contact the restaurant in advance. The Coeliac Society website contains further examples of questions to ask the chef, as well as the most important information on gluten-free diets.

9. WHAT DO I DO IF I'M IN HOSPITAL?

Hospital kitchens are equipped for various diets. If you have planned a stay in hospital, explain your needs to the staff beforehand. However, mistakes can still be made, so you must always check every meal. If you are taken to hospital in an emergency, make sure you or your family inform someone of your condition immediately.

THE DIAGNOSIS

POSSIBILITIES AND CERTAINTIES

Reliable diagnoses require an antibody test as well as a biopsy. The diagnosis is only truly definite if both results match. If the test results differ, other possible causes should also be examined. If the intestinal mucosa displays damage despite a negative blood test result, a gluten-free diet should be maintained, and a follow-up biopsy should be taken at a later date as a precaution.

The body's own immune system recognises gluten components as antigens, and produces protective/defensive antibodies, which can be detected in a blood test. Both the IgA antibodies and the IgG antibodies should be tested, as two percent of all coeliac sufferers are IgA deficient. In addition to the gliadin antibody test, transglutaminase antibodies are now also tested, because their levels are typically elevated in those suffering from coeliac disease.

To take a biopsy of the small intestine, an endoscope or biopsy capsule is fed into the upper section of the small intestine through the mouth. This allows the doctor to take small samples of the surface of the patient's intestine. The procedure can be performed under local anaesthetic so it is not painful, and it is straightforward. Patients are usually advised to come accompanied by another person.

Both examinations should be performed during an acute stage of the disease when the patient is experiencing symptoms in order to ensure reliable diagnosis. If a gluten-free diet was adopted after the initial diagnostic evaluation, the results of the examination will be unreliable. Annual check-ups can be conducted at a later date as a precaution.

POSSIBLE COMORBID DISEASES

> diabetes mellitus
> rheumatic disorders
> renal disorders
> Crohn's disease/colitis ulcerosa
> skin diseases
> gastritis
> lactose intolerance
> allergies

BIOPSY	BLOOD TEST	DIAGNOSIS	TREATMENT
positive	positive	reliably positive	gluten-free diet
negative	negative	reliably negative	no gluten-free diet
positive	negative	possible coeliac disease with IgA deficiency	IgG detection gluten-free diet follow-up biopsy
negative	positive	possible hypersensitivity without acute symptoms	no gluten-free diet follow-up biopsy

MY CHILD
HAS COELIAC DISEASE

WHAT SHOULD I DO?

Putting infants and small children on gluten-free diets is not usually any hassle. It only becomes problematic if the child notices differences between his/her gluten-free food and the prohibited "normal" food. To ensure they do not feel like an outsider within the family, it is very important that the whole family eats gluten-free foods. You should explain the need for gluten-free eating to your child's friends, and especially to their parents. Teachers at school must similarly be informed. It is important for the issue to be handled in a simple, honest and objective manner. The child should not be made to feel different in either a positive or negative way.

LUNCHTIME AT SCHOOL

Give the teachers, carers and lunchtime supervisors all the details they need for understanding coeliac disease, and explain the consequences of eating the wrong foods to ensure the gluten-free diet is taken seriously. Be sure to note when there is any change of staff and always inform them personally. If the food is prepared at the school itself, there is a risk that your child's needs may not be able to be taken into account, and also that mistakes will be made. As a precaution, your child should therefore always bring food from home that you have prepared yourself. If the school's food is supplied by a large-scale catering establishment, contact the head office and ask whether gluten-free food is an option.

CHILDREN'S BIRTHDAY PARTIES

If a child with coeliac disease is invited to a birthday party, speak to their friend's parents beforehand, and give your child home-made gluten-free cakes and biscuits instead to take with them. Only assume there will be gluten-free food if you can be sure the parents are familiar with gluten-free food preparation, and so all precautions will be taken.

You can bake this chocolate cake for a child's birthday party without any problems: Serves 12: 250 g (8 oz) chocolate, 250 g (8 oz) butter, 150 g (5 oz) sugar, 8 egg yolks, 5 egg whites, 160 g (5⅓ oz) ground hazelnuts

Melt the chocolate over hot water. Cut the butter into pieces, and mix with the sugar until frothy. Stir in the egg yolks. Add the melted chocolate. Beat the egg whites until stiff, carefully folding in the hazelnuts. Then fold the egg white and hazelnut mixture into the butter mixture. Pour the batter into a greased cake tin and bake for 35 minutes at 180°C (355°F)/160 °C fanforced.

SCHOOL TRIPS AND EXCURSIONS

Give your child enough food for the excursion to ensure they are not reliant on other food sources. For school trips, you must make sure the kitchen can prepare gluten-free meals. Ask the staff in person ahead of time, whether this is possible. Give children gluten-free bread, pastries and sweets to take with them instead.

GENERAL QUESTIONS

1. IS THERE ANYTHING THAT I SHOULD BE PARTICULARLY CAREFUL OF DURING THE EARLY STAGES?

If you are experiencing difficulties digesting fats, switch to easily digestible MCT (medium-chain triglycerides) fats. Follow the general principles of healthy eating, and incorporate as many dietary fibres into your diet as possible. Avoid foods which cause bloating such as cabbage, onions, leek and legumes.

2. CAN I TRUST THE INFORMATION ON THE FOOD LABELS?

In most countries, all foods and ingredients capable of triggering allergies and intolerances must be declared on the label. This means that gluten-containing food and food with glutenous additives must be labelled, and the specific sources stated. It is the ready-made meals and processed foods that you should pay particular attention to, studying each label in detail.

3. WHAT IS "GLUTEN-FREE WHEAT STARCH"?

Wheat-starch production involves primary starch or "A starch" containing up to 0.5% protein and secondary starch or "B-starch" containing up to 5% protein. Secondary starch is definitely not suitable for a gluten-free diet. General foods with low starch content may contain primary starch. Foods can only be labelled gluten-free if they contain no detectable gluten (0–5 ppm, preferably 0), no oats and no malted cereals containing gluten in their products.

4. ARE THERE ANY SUBSIDIES AVAILABLE FOR PURCHASING THE DIETARY FOODS I NEED TO EAT?

In general, health insurance funds do not pay any subsidies for dietary foods, but you should still clarify this with your individual insurer.

5. CAN I DONATE BLOOD IF I HAVE COELIAC DISEASE?

As there are no national or international guidelines for donating blood, your GP should decide in your particular case whether you are able to do so or not. In principle, coeliac disease does not constitute a reason for ineligibility, provided no acute symptoms exist. If they do, donating blood is generally not permitted.

6. WHAT IS LACTOSE INTOLERANCE?

Lactose intolerance is an intolerance to the milk sugar known as lactose. Acute cases of coeliac disease are often simultaneously associated with lactose intolerance, as the small intestine no longer produces the necessary lactase enzyme. Lactose intolerance can be diagnosed by a hydrogen breath test or blood test. If the result is positive, all milk products and food containing lactose must be avoided. The book *Great Healthy Food Lactose-Free* by Knox and Lowman provides more information and suitable recipes.

7. WHAT ARE THE SYMPTOMS OF DERMATITIS HERPETIFORMIS OR DUHRING'S DISEASE?

D.h.D. or Duhring's disease is a skin disease often associated with coeliac disease. In acute cases, itchiness is followed by blisters (elbows, knees and head). A skin test can provide a reliable diagnosis. If the result is positive, the patient should also be checked for coeliac disease, as this skin disorder is often a sign of dormant coeliac disease. Duhring's disease can be treated with medication – you should weigh up the pros and cons. Iodine is a frequent trigger, so sufferers must be sure to remove both gluten and iodine from their diet.

INITIAL STEPS
AFTER DIAGNOSIS

MOVE FORWARD PURPOSEFULLY

It is quite normal to feel scared, uncertain and frustrated in the first few days after diagnosis, but try to be grateful that the cause of your symptoms has been identified and can now be treated. Look for a self-help group near you, and then do your best to move forward purposefully and methodically.

- Involve all the members of your household. Inform your acquaintances and relatives, especially if the coeliac sufferer is a child. The more people know about it the easier it will be for you to stick to the diet.
- Clean all kitchen utensils, especially toasters, bread baskets and bread cutters, or buy a second set of new ones.
- Replace all everyday items made of wood, as glutenous residue may have been deposited in the notches and grooves of cutting boards and wooden spoons.
- Always prepare gluten-free food separately from food containing gluten, preferably making the gluten-free dishes first. Your family may be happy to share a gluten-free diet with you.
- Clean all cooking, roasting, baking and frying utensils after use.
- In general, avoid using the same kitchen utensils when preparing glutenous and gluten-free food.

- Use different, preferably labelled dishcloths, tea towels and hand towels for gluten-free and gluten-containing items.
- Do not re-use deep-frying fat in which glutenous foods may have been prepared beforehand.
- Always store glutenous and gluten-free food items separately, in separate cupboards if possible, and clearly label all storage containers to avoid any possible mix-up.
- Always make sure storage containers, such as jars or tins, previously containing glutenous rice are cleaned thoroughly.
- Check all stored foods, such as spices, stocks and teas, for gluten. Throw out any that you are not sure about, or use them only in dishes for people without coeliac disease.
- Label baking dishes, baking sheets and baking machine trays for gluten-free cakes and pastries, or use baking paper.
- Always store gluten-free bread separately from normal bread.
- Use different bread baskets and toasters for gluten-free and gluten-containing breads.
- Always wash the bread knife carefully, or use two different knives.

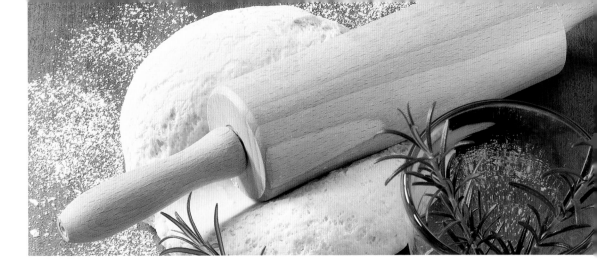

AVOID HIDDEN DIET TRAPS

- Carefully study the Ingredient List published by your local Coeliac Society. Take it with you when you go shopping for food.
- Learn how to interpret food labels, and take sufficient time to read all the nutritional information on foods when doing your grocery shopping.
- Find out which gluten-free foods are available at the stores that are conveniently located for you to access.
- Expand your shopping routines and habits to include health food shops and organic food shops. Try purchasing gluten-free ingredients for your home cooking from specialist suppliers via the Internet.
- Check non-food items also, for example medications, toothpaste, dental hygiene products and lipsticks, and replace these if necessary.
- Food not labelled as gluten-free may be contaminated with traces of gluten.
- Make sure no grains are ground at the health food shop, as its mill is bound to have been used to grind grains containing gluten.
- When buying your own grain mill, make sure this is only used to grind gluten-free grains.

THE FOLLOWING ITEMS MAY CONTAIN HIDDEN GLUTEN

- > medication
- > vitamin formulations
- > lipsticks, lip-care products
- > toothpaste, oral hygiene products
- > spice mixtures
- > "... products"
- > "light" products
- > ice cream
- > fruit slices
- > tea mixtures
- > malt products
- > additives
- > flavouring agents
- > colouring agents
- > play dough/plasticine

Due to its close botanical relationship with oats, wild rice was long suspected of also containing gluten, but latest findings show otherwise. It adds a different colour to dishes and a pleasantly nutty flavour. However, you will need to cook wild rice dishes for longer.

GLUTEN-FREE BAKING

DO I HAVE TO BAKE MY OWN BREAD?

If there is nowhere for you to purchase fresh gluten-free bread, the only way to be on the safe side is to bake your own bread. Homemade bread is usually tastier anyway, and it will certainly be cheaper than buying gluten-free bread. You can try out different recipes and some unusual ingredients and vary them according to your tastes.

IS IT WORTH BUYING A BREAD-MAKER?

Bread is baked in an oven with top/bottom heating or in a fan-forced oven, although a bread-maker can make this job much easier. The advantages of a bread-maker are the optimised kneading phase and baking process, and the fact that nice fresh bread can be produced within a short space of time. Make sure you use it only for gluten-free bread.

WHICH FLOURS CAN I COMBINE?

Maize flour, rice flour and buckwheat flour can be mixed with potato starch or cornflour (cornstarch), carob bean gum (locust bean gum) or xanthan gum. The buckwheat flour can be substituted with amaranth flour, chestnut flour, chickpea flour or quinoa flour. These special flours are available at health food shops.

WHAT CAN I USE AS A BINDING AGENT, AND WHAT WILL MAKE THE DOUGH LIGHTER AND FLUFFIER?

Guar gum, carob bean gum (locust bean gum), xanthan gum or arrowroot flour are all suitable binding agents. Use fruit vinegar to make the dough lighter and fluffier. Simply stir 1–3 tsp into the dough and continue as before.

WHAT MAKES THE BREAD DOUGH SMOOTHER?

So-called psyllium plantago is ideal for improving bread's preparation and baking properties, as it has a particular tendency to swell. This allows it to absorb a lot of liquid and retain it better in gluten-free pastries and breads. Psyllium is the seed capsule of plantain. It has only recently started being used in gluten-free cooking, but is now a common component in some ready-made flours due to its favourable properties.

HOW DO I USE PSYLLIUM?

Simply stir 1–2 tsp psyllium into the liquid required for making the bread dough, leave to swell for 10 minutes, add to the dough, then continue as normal. Ground psyllium may be sold under the name of psyllium fibre husk, but you can also buy it whole (unground) from pharmacies and grind it yourself in a dedicated mill.

WHAT MAKES BREAD DOUGH RISE BETTER?

All ingredients should be at room temperature. Only prove the dough once. Briefly heat the oven to 50°C (120°F) , then switch it off. Place the dough in a bowl covered with a damp cloth, and put this into the oven. On hot summer days, when outside temperatures are high, the standing time can be shortened; it can be prolonged in winter.

HOW CAN I SHAPE GLUTEN-FREE PASTRIES AND BAKED PRODUCTS?

Bake the bread in an oblong cake or loaf tin or in a special round or oval baking tin. Bread rolls can be moulded with moistened hands and then dipped in sesame seeds, poppy seeds or sunflower seeds. The dough can also be moulded into scrolls, rings, pretzel shapes or flat cakes.

HOW DOES THE BREAD GET A NICE CRUST?

To ensure the bread forms a thick crust, coat the dough with some lukewarm water, coffee, lukewarm milk or egg yolk whisked in oil before baking. Coating it with egg white or egg yolk will also give the bread a lovely shiny surface.

Place a small heatproof bowl of water in the oven along with the bread dough as you are baking it to prevent it from drying out too much.

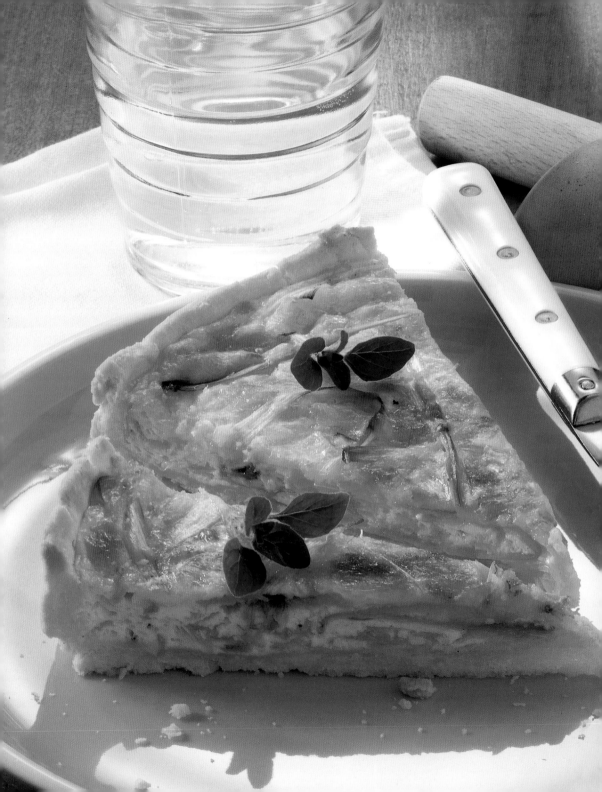

THE RECIPES

MAKING GLUTEN-FREE COOKING AND BAKING ENJOYABLE

Are you still finding it hard to switch to a gluten-free diet because you don't know which substitute products are suitable for cooking and baking?

Don't worry; this chapter will show you how to conjure up the best meals, even without gluten. The manufacturer information in the ingredient lists will make it easier for you to choose products. All recipes are guaranteed to be gluten-free, varied and, most importantly, tasty so you can enjoy them without worrying. The range of soups and sauces, baked items, sweet treats, delicious cakes, as well as mains, will soon convince you and your family that you can do without gluten when cooking.

Vegetable Soup with polenta gnocchi

SERVES 4

350 ml (12 fl oz/1½ cups) vegetable
stock

140 g (4½ oz) polenta

salt, pepper, nutmeg

1 egg

1 tbsp cream

3 tbsp chopped fresh herbs
(e.g. parsley, chives)

1 litre (32 fl oz/4 cups) vegetable
or meat stock

PREPARATION about 35 mins

1. Bring the vegetable stock to the boil. Sprinkle in the polenta and bring back to the boil. Leave to simmer for about 5 minutes, stirring constantly. Turn off the heat and leave the polenta to rise for 15 minutes.

2. Bring plenty of salted water to the boil in a large saucepan.

3. Season the polenta mixture with salt, pepper and nutmeg to taste and leave to cool a little. Stir together the egg and the cream, then stir this and the herbs into the polenta mixture.

4. Using two teaspoons, shape small gnocchi and place them into the boiling salted water. Leave to cook for a few minutes until the gnocchi rise to the surface. Serve in hot vegetable or meat stock, sprinkled with 1 tablespoon chopped herbs.

VARIATION

Stir 4 tablespoons Parmesan into the gnocchi mixture to give the soup a cheesy note.

TIP

You can make the vegetable stock yourself, using fresh vegetables, but you could also use instant vegetable soup instead.

NUTRITIONAL VALUES PER PORTION:

220 Cal • 5 g protein • 6 g fat • 33 g carbohydrate

Cream of Mushroom Soup

SERVES 4

750 ml (24 fl oz/3 cups)
vegetable stock

1 onion

200 g (6½ oz) fresh mushrooms

2 tbsp rapeseed oil

3 tbsp gluten-free plain flour

50 ml (2 fl oz/¼ cup) milk

50 ml (2 fl oz/¼ cup) cream

50 ml (2 fl oz/¼ cup) white wine
(alternatively 50 ml 2 fl oz/
¼ cup extra vegetable stock)

1 tbsp lemon juice

salt, nutmeg

freshly ground white pepper

2 tbsp snipped chives

PREPARATION about 20 mins

1. Bring the vegetable stock to the boil. Peel and dice the onion. Wipe, then slice the mushrooms. Reserve some mushroom slices for the garnish.

2. Heat the oil in a large saucepan. Add the onion and sauté until transparent. Add the mushroom slices and fry for 2 minutes. Dust with the flour and continue frying for another 2 minutes, stirring constantly. Pour in the hot vegetable stock and simmer for 6–8 minutes over a low temperature.

3. Add the milk and the cream to the soup and purée using a food processor or hand-held blender. Season to taste with wine, lemon juice, salt, nutmeg and pepper. Sprinkle with the reserved mushroom slices and the chives. Serve immediately.

VARIATION

To make a cream of vegetable soup, simply use cauliflower or broccoli florets, zucchini (courgette) dice or slices of fennel to replace the mushroom slices in this recipe.

NUTRITIONAL VALUES PER PORTION:

165 Cal • 2 g protein • 9 g fat • 15 g carbohydrate

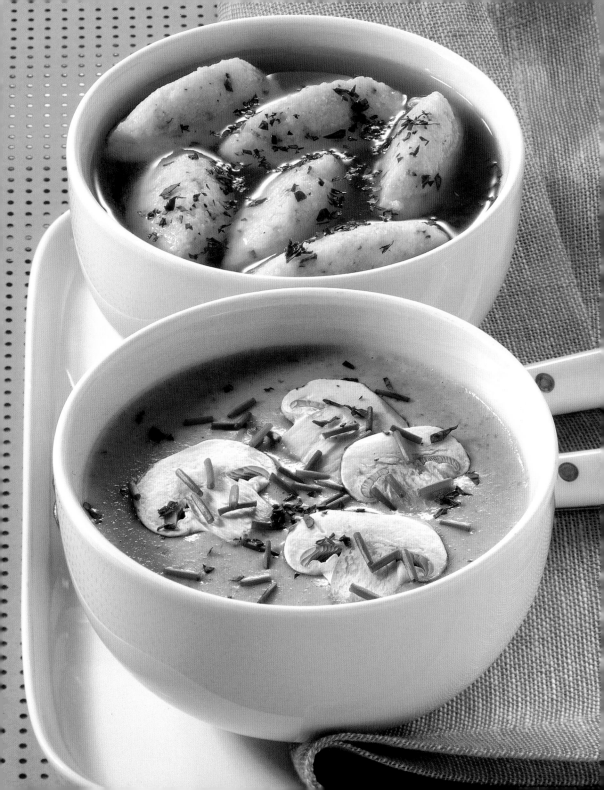

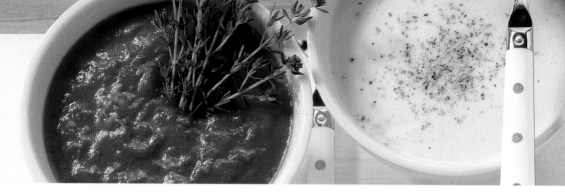

Tasty Tomato Sauce

SERVES 4

1 onion

1-2 garlic cloves

2 tbsp olive oil

400 g (13 oz) tinned chopped
   tomatoes

3 tbsp tomato paste (purée)

salt, pepper

3 tbsp red wine (if desired)

5 tbsp cream

1 tbsp chopped fresh herbs
   (e.g. oregano, thyme, basil)

PREPARATION about 30 mins

1. Peel the onion and the garlic, then chop into small dice. Heat the oil in a saucepan, add the onion and garlic dice and fry, stirring, until transparent.

2. Stir in the chopped tomatoes and their juice and simmer briefly. Add the tomato paste. Season with salt and pepper, then simmer for about 10 minutes over a low temperature.

3. Add the red wine and simmer for another 5 minutes. Before serving, stir in the cream and the herbs. This sauce is perfect with freshly cooked pasta.

VARIATIONS

For a different version you could also add 200 g (6½ oz) fried minced beef or 200 g (6½ oz) finely chopped fried vegetable strips, for example carrot, leek, celery or zucchini (courgette).

NUTRITIONAL VALUES PER PORTION:

140 Cal • 2 g protein • 11 g fat • 5 g carbohydrate

Béchamel Sauce

SERVES 4

2 tbsp clarified butter (ghee)

40 g (1½ oz) gluten-free plain flour

200 ml (7 fl oz/¾ cup)
   vegetable stock

200 ml (7 fl oz/¾ cup) milk

salt, nutmeg

2 tbsp cream

PREPARATION about 20 mins

1. Melt the clarified butter in a saucepan, then stir in the flour. Add the stock and the milk. Stir vigorously so that the flour doesn't clump.

2. Season with salt and nutmeg. Bring to the boil. Now add the cream but do not allow the Béchamel sauce to come back to the boil again.

VARIATIONS

Sprinkle the sauce with some chopped parsley and it will go particularly well with parsley and cream potatoes.

Use this sauce together with tomato sauce to make lasagne.

Stir 50 g (1²/₃ oz) grated cheese into the sauce.

NUTRITIONAL VALUES PER PORTION:

120 Cal • 2 g protein • 10 g fat • 12 g carbohydrate

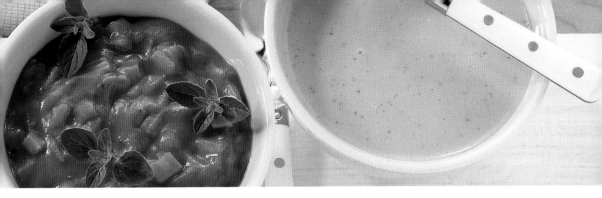

Spicy Barbecue Sauce

SERVES 6

2 spring onions (shallots)

3 garlic cloves

1 stick celery

2 tbsp olive oil

6 tbsp tomato sauce

6 tbsp tomato paste (purée)

2 tbsp balsamic vinegar

1 tbsp Dijon mustard

salt, pepper

1 tbsp chopped fresh herbs
  (e.g. thyme, oregano, basil)

PREPARATION about 30 mins

1. Trim the spring onions, peel the garlic, then finely dice both. Wash the celery and pull off any hard strings; finely chop. Heat the oil in a saucepan. Add onion and garlic, fry until transparent. Add the celery and sauté briefly.

2. Add the tomato sauce, tomato paste, vinegar, mustard and 150 ml (5 fl oz/¾ cup) water, then simmer the sauce for about 20 minutes. Season with salt, pepper and herbs.

TIP

In a screw-top jar the sauce will keep for at least 2 weeks when chilled.
If you fill the sauce into a screw-top bottle that has been sterilised first (washed out with boiling water), the sauce will keep for up to 4 months as long as the bottle has not been opened.

NUTRITIONAL VALUES PER PORTION:

60 Cal • 1 g protein • 3 g fat • 7 g carbohydrate

Creamy Curry Sauce

SERVES 4

1 small onion

2 tbsp olive oil

30 g (1 oz) gluten-free plain flour

3 tsp curry powder

250 ml (8 fl oz/1 cup) chicken stock

salt, pepper, sugar, garlic powder

200 g (6½ oz) cream, 1 egg yolk

PREPARATION about 20 mins

1. Peel and dice the onion. Heat the oil in a non-stick saucepan and fry the onion dice until transparent. Stir in the flour and the curry powder. Pour in the chicken stock and bring to the boil, stirring.

2. Season the sauce to taste with salt, pepper and garlic powder. Stir together the cream and the egg yolk, then add. Heat the sauce but do not bring it to the boil again.

VARIATION

Refine the curry sauce with 3 tablespoons each of small pineapple and peach dice.

NUTRITIONAL VALUES PER PORTION:

258 Cal • 2 g protein • 23 g fat • 10 g carbohydrate

Gnocchi with Parmesan

SERVES 4

800 g (1lb 10 oz) unpeeled, cooked
  floury potatoes (from the day
  before if possible)
50 g (1²/₃ oz) low-fat cream cheese
1 egg
150 g (5 oz) freshly grated Parmesan
70 g (2½ oz) gluten-free plain flour
80 g (2¾ oz) fine polenta, plus some
  for dusting
salt, nutmeg
butter for greasing
30 g (1 oz) butter

PREPARATION about 1 hr
BAKING about 10 mins

1. Preheat the oven to 200°C (390°F)/180°C (355°F) fan-forced. Bring salted water to the boil in a large saucepan. Slip off the skins of the cooked potatoes, then push them through a potato ricer. Combine with the cream cheese, egg, half the Parmesan, the flour and the polenta and quickly work into a dough. Season with salt and nutmeg.

2. Sprinkle a baking board with the polenta, then shape the dough into finger-thick rolls. Cut the rolls into 2–3 cm (¾–1¼ in) lengths. Lightly flatten each piece with the back of a fork.

3. Place the gnocchi into the boiling salted water and leave to cook over a medium heat until they rise to the surface. Lift them out with a slotted spoon and leave to drain a little.

4. Lightly grease an ovenproof baking dish, then place the gnocchi into the dish. Sprinkle with the remaining Parmesan and the butter pats. Bake in the oven for 10 minutes. The gnocchi are delicious served with tomato sauce and a green or mixed salad.

VARIATION
GNOCCHI ON A BED OF SPINACH

1 small onion
2 garlic cloves
2 tbsp olive oil
450 g (15 oz) frozen leaf spinach
salt, pepper, nutmeg
3 tbsp crème fraîche
150 g (5 oz) freshly grated Parmesan cheese
butter for greasing

Preheat the oven to 220°C (430°F)/200°C (390°F) fan-forced. Prepare the gnocchi following the recipe until the end of Step 3. Grease the dish. Peel onion and garlic, then finely dice both. Heat the oil in a large frying pan and sauté the onion and the garlic until transparent. Add the spinach and continue sautéing over a low heat, until it is completely defrosted. Season to taste with salt, pepper and nutmeg. Stir in the crème fraîche. Transfer the spinach mixture to the dish. Place the gnocchi on top and sprinkle with the Parmesan cheese. Bake in the oven for 15-20 minutes until golden.

NUTRITIONAL VALUES PER PORTION:
480 Cal • 23 g protein • 19 g fat • 54 g carbohydrate

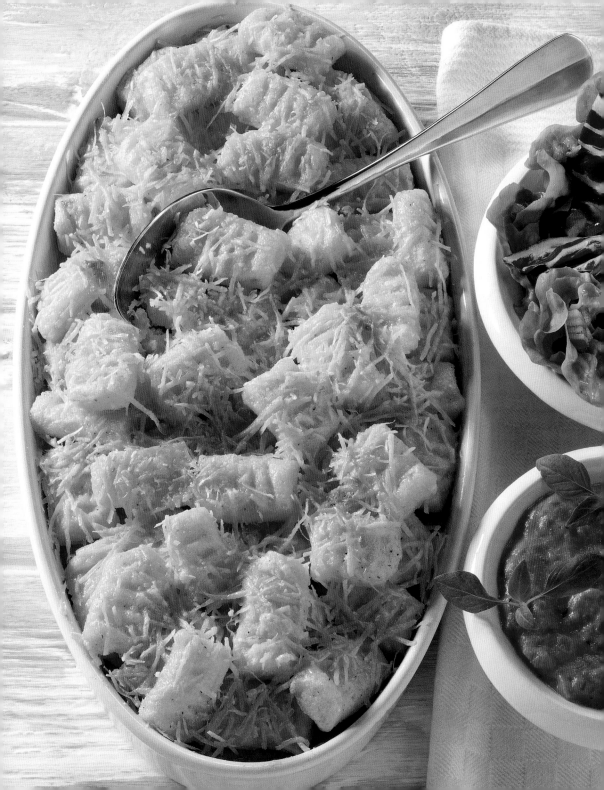

Cheesy Polenta Bake

SERVES 4

200 g (6½ oz) gluten-free
    plain flour

50 g (1²⁄₃ oz) fine polenta

3 eggs

1 tbsp oil

1 tsp salt

1 large onion

1 tbsp clarified butter

butter for greasing

150 g (5 oz) grated Emmental cheese

PREPARATION about 30 mins

RESTING about 20 mins

BAKING about 10 mins

1. Stir together the polenta, eggs, oil and salt to make a doughy batter. Add some more water depending on the size of the eggs – the consistency should be that of a firm sponge. Leave the batter to rest for about 20 minues (covered, at room temperature) so the polenta can expand.

2. Meanwhile bring salted water to the boil in a large saucepan. Press the batter, a portion at a time, through a potato ricer – you will need to push quite firmly. Place the dumplings, a few at a time, into the boiling water, bring back to the boil, then lift out with a slotted spoon. Drain in a sieve.

3. Preheat the oven to 220°C (430°F)/200°C (390°F) fan-forced (middle shelf). Peel and finely dice the onion. Melt the clarified butter in a frying pan and sauté the onion until it is golden. Lightly grease an ovenproof baking dish.

4. Alternate layers of the hot dumplings, the cheese and the fried onion in the gratin dish. Bake in the oven for 10 minutes. If you don't want the crust to be too crisp, cover the top with aluminium foil. A mixed salad goes well with this dish.

VARIATION

Fry 100 g (3⅓ oz) bacon dice together with the onion. It will make this a hearty main course meal.

TIP

The dumplings are well-suited for freezing. To serve, bake in the oven at 200°C (390°F)/180°C (355°F) fan-forced (middle shelf) for about 10 minutes.

NUTRITIONAL VALUES PER PORTION:
505 Cal • 18 g protein • 25 g fat • 52 g carbohydrate

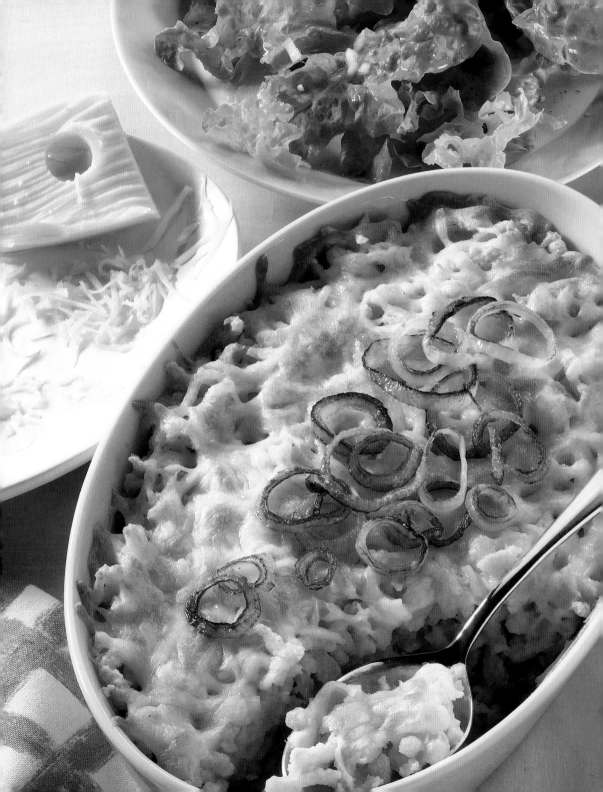

Penne with zucchini sauce

SERVES 4

1 onion

2 garlic cloves

400 g (13 oz) zucchini (courgettes)

4 tbsp olive oil

400 g (13 oz) tinned chopped
tomatoes

100 g (3⅓ oz) cream

salt, pepper

400 g (13 oz) gluten-free penne

50 g (1⅔ oz) freshly grated
Parmesan

2 tbsp freshly chopped basil

PREPARATION about 30 mins

1. Peel and finely dice the onion and the garlic. Wash the zucchini and cut them into thin strips. Heat the oil in a frying pan and sauté the onion and garlic dice until transparent. Add the zucchini strips and fry briefly. Add the chopped tomatoes with their juice and leave to simmer for about 5 minutes over a low temperature.

2. Stir in the cream, season the sauce with salt and pepper to taste. Cook the penne according to packet instructions in boiling salted water until al dente (firm to the bite). Drain. Serve portions with the sauce and sprinkle with Parmesan and chopped basil.

VARIATION

Add 50 g (1⅔ oz) diced ham or prosciutto to the sauce to turn this into a heartier main course dish.

NUTRITIONAL VALUES PER PORTION:

610 Cal • 20 g protein • 23 g fat • 81 g carbohydrate

Spaghetti carbonara

SERVES 4

1 bunch parsley

80 g (2¾ oz) pancetta or
streaky bacon

2 garlic cloves

500 g (1 lb) gluten-free spaghetti

40 g (1½ oz) butter

125 g (4 oz) cream

3 eggs

3 egg yolks

60 g (2 oz) grated Parmesan

salt, pepper

PREPARATION about 30 mins

1. Wash the parsley, shake it dry, then finely chop it. Dice the bacon and peel the garlic.

2. Cook the spaghetti according to packet instructions until al dente (firm to the bite). Heat the butter in a frying pan, sauté the garlic cloves and remove them from the pan after 3 minutes. Place the bacon into the same pan and sauté for about 5 minutes. Add the cream and briefly bring the sauce to the boil.

3. In a bowl, combine the eggs and the egg yolks with the chopped parsley and the grated Parmesan. Drain the spaghetti. Add to the hot bacon and cream mixture, then pour over the stirred eggs and thoroughly combine. Season with salt and pepper and serve immediately.

TIP

Pre-warm the bowl with a little boiling water.

NUTRITIONAL VALUES PER PORTION:

925 Cal • 32 g protein • 46 g fat • 96 g carbohydrate

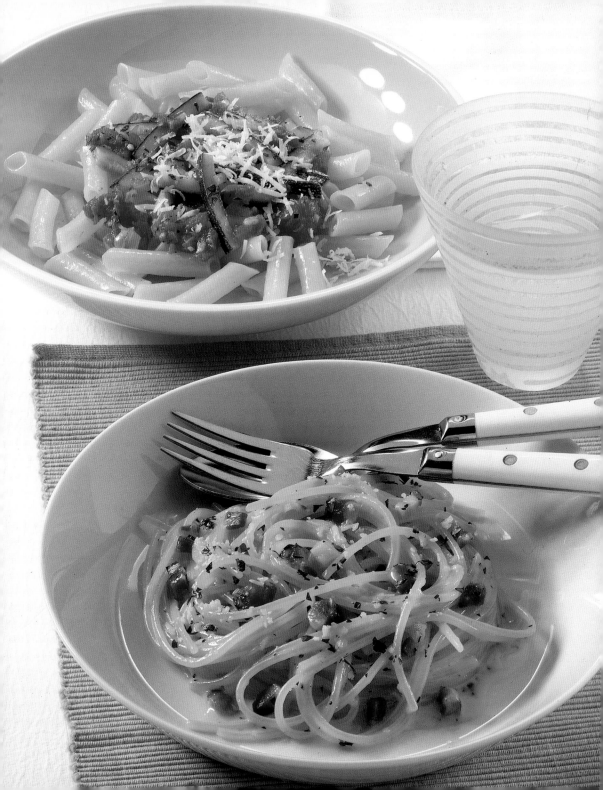

Lasagne

SERVES 4-6

double quantity Tomato Sauce with
  vegetables or mince
  (see page 28, variations)
1 quantity Béchamel Sauce
  (see page 28)
1 pack gluten-free lasagne
  sheets (250 g/8 oz)
150 g (5 oz) freshly grated Parmesan
30 g (1 oz) cold butter
olive oil for greasing
PREPARATION about 2 hrs
BAKING about 40 mins

1. Prepare the sauces according to the recipes (see page 28).

2. In a large saucepan bring plenty of salted water to the boil. Add a dash of oil and cook the lasagne sheets in two batches for 5 minutes each. Lift out with a slotted spoon and place the sheets side by side on a moistened platter or board (do not place them on top of each other or they will stick together).

3. Preheat the oven to 220°C (430°F)/200°C (390°F) fan-forced (middle shelf). Grease a baking dish with olive oil, then cover the base of the dish with 2–3 tablespoons tomato sauce. Add 2–3 tablespoons béchamel sauce, stir, sprinkle with a little Parmesan. Cover with a layer of lasagne sheets, then spread again with the sauces. Repeat until all the lasagne sheets and the sauces have been used up.

4. Sprinkle the final layer of sauces with the remaining cheese and place the butter in small pats on top. Bake the lasagne in the oven for about 35–40 minutes. Leave to rest for a few mnutes before serving. A green salad goes well with this delicious pasta dish.

TIP

You can prepare the lasagne the day before and leave it covered with foil in the fridge until you are ready to bake it. You could also freeze the lasagne and bake it in the oven at 220°C (430°F)/200°C (390°F) fan-forced (middle shelf) for about 35-40 minutes.

VARIATION

If you have no lasagne sheets to hand, simply use any other gluten-free pasta instead.

NUTRITIONAL VALUES PER PORTION:
1010 Cal • 49 g protein • 50 g fat • 87 g carbohydrate

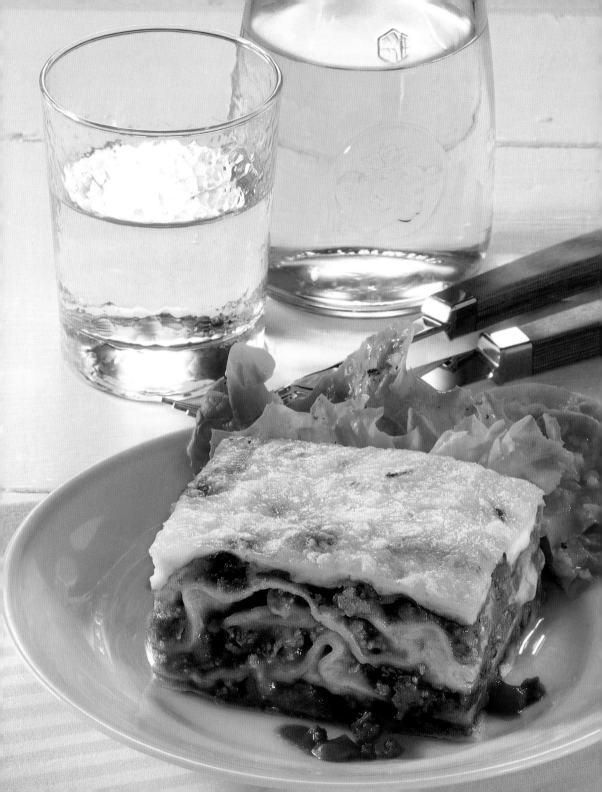

Meaty Pasta Parcels

SERVES 4
FOR THE DOUGH
300 g (10 oz) gluten-free plain flour
1 tsp salt
1 tsp psyllium (fibre husk)
3 eggs
1 tbsp rapeseed oil
FOR THE FILLING
1 onion
½ bunch parsley
1 tbsp oil
50 g (1⅔ oz) salami
300 g (10 oz) lean minced beef
1 egg
1 tbsp gluten-free breadcrumbs
salt, pepper
1 egg white for brushing
1 onion
2 tbsp butter
PREPARATION about 1 hr
RESTING about 20 mins

1. Combine the flour with the salt and the psyllium. Knead into a firm dough together with the eggs and the oil, adding about 2–3 tablespoons cold water if needed. Wrap the dough in cling film; chill for about 20 minutes.

2. Peel and dice the onion. Wash and shake dry the parsley, then finely chop it. Heat the oil and sauté the onion and the parsley until the onion is transparent, then leave to cool a little. Very finely dice the salami and knead it together with the minced beef, egg and breadcrumbs. Season with salt and pepper. Mix in the cooled parsley and onion mixture.

3. In a large saucepan, bring plenty of salted water to the boil. Roll out the pasta dough as thinly as possible, then cut it into squares of about 10 cm (4 in). Place 1 teaspoon of the filling on one half of each of the squares. Brush the edge of the dough squares with a little egg white, then fold the other half on top. With a fork press the edges so they stick together.

4. Place the pasta parcels into the boiling salted water and briefly bring to the boil, then reduce the heat and simmer for about 8 minutes. Meanwhile peel and finely dice the onion. Melt the butter and fry the onion until a golden yellow. Pour the onion butter over the pasta parcels before serving. Serve with a lukewarm potato salad and a green salad.

VARIATION

For a delicious variation, mix 50 g (1⅔ oz) chopped spinach into the meat filling for the pasta parcels.

TIP

The pasta parcels are well suited to freezing raw. To prepare them, place the frozen parcels straight into the boiling salted water, bring to the boil once and then allow to simmer for about 10 minutes.

NUTRITIONAL VALUES PER PORTION:
655 Cal • 29 g protein • 31 g fat • 67 g carbohydrate

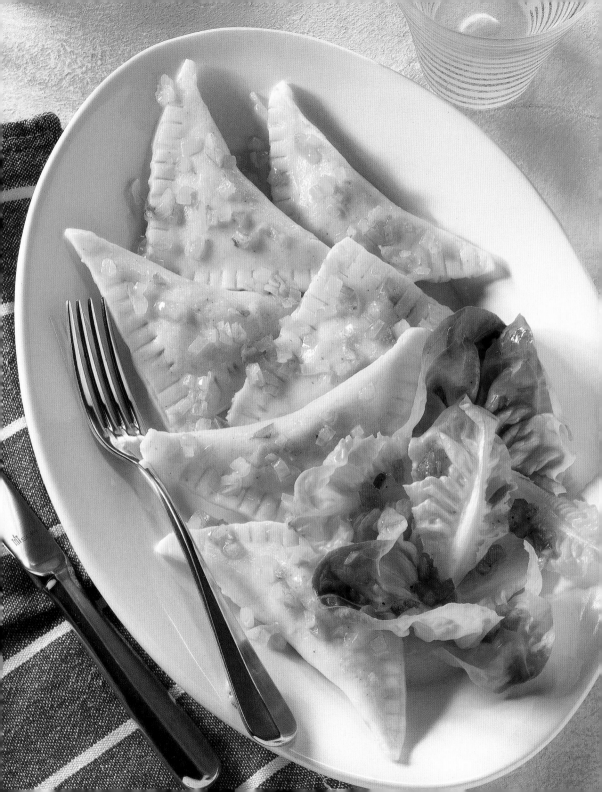

Pickled Beef Roast with bread dumplings

SERVES 4–6

FOR THE MARINADE
(1 WEEK BEFORE COOKING)

330 ml (11 fl oz/1½ cups)
dry red wine

330 ml (11 fl oz/1½ cups)
wine vinegar

330 ml (11 fl oz/1½ cups) water

1 onion

1 bay leaf

2 cloves

10 black peppercorns

1 kg (2 lb 4 oz) beef roast

FOR THE ROAST

3 carrots

mustard, salt, pepper

6 tbsp rapeseed oil

2 tbsp redcurrant jelly

2 tbsp cornflour (cornstarch)

3 tbsp crème fraîche

FOR THE BREAD DUMPLINGS

400 g (13 oz) gluten-free
white bread

150 ml (5 fl oz/¾ cup)
lukewarm milk

1 small onion

½ bunch parsley

2 tbsp rapeseed oil

50 g (1²/₃ oz) diced bacon

1 large egg

salt, nutmeg

gluten-free breadcrumbs for
the work surface

PREPARATION about 2 hrs

MARINATING about 1 week

1. In a large saucepan or bowl, stir together the red wine, the vinegar and the water. Peel the onion, then cut into rings. Add to the red wine mixture together with the bay leaf, the cloves and the peppercorns. Place the beef in the marinade mixture, cover and leave to marinate in the refrigerator for 1 week.

2. On the day of preparation, peel the carrots, quarter them lengthways and cut the quarters into sticks of approximately 3 cm (1¼ in). Lift the beef and the onion rings out of the marinade. Drain the onion rings and pat the meat dry with kitchen paper. Rub the roast all over with mustard and season it generously with salt and pepper.

3. Heat the oil in a large braising pot and fry the meat all over on high heat. Add the carrots and onion rings, then braise on medium heat for 2–3 minutes.

4. Add the redcurrant jelly, then pour in one-third of the marinade. Cover and braise for about 1 hour, adding more of the marinade from time to time.

5. To make the bread dumplings, dry out the white bread on a baking tray in the oven at 50°C for about 30 minutes. Cut the bread into small dice, pour over the lukewarm milk and leave to soak for 10 minutes.

6. Peel and dice the onion. Wash and shake dry, then finely chop the parsley. Heat the oil in a frying pan, add the onion, the bacon and the parsley, and fry until the onion is translucent. Leave the mixture to cool a little.

7. In a large saucepan, bring plenty of salted water to the boil. Knead the bacon and onion with the egg mixture into the bread mixture. Season with salt and nutmeg. If the dough is too moist, knead in some gluten-free breadcrumbs. With moistened hands, shape the mixture into 8 dumplings. Lower them into the boiling salted water and simmer over low heat for 15 minutes.

8. Lift the meat out of the pot and keep warm. Pour off the cooking juices through a sieve or purée them, then bring to the boil. Dissolve the cornflour in a little water, then stir into the simmering gravy and bring to the boil. Stir in the crème fraîche.

9. Lift out the dumplings with a slotted spoon. Cut the roast into slices and serve with the gravy and the bread dumplings.

NUTRITIONAL VALUES PER PORTION:
860 Cal • 49 g protein • 37 g fat • 79 g carbohydrate

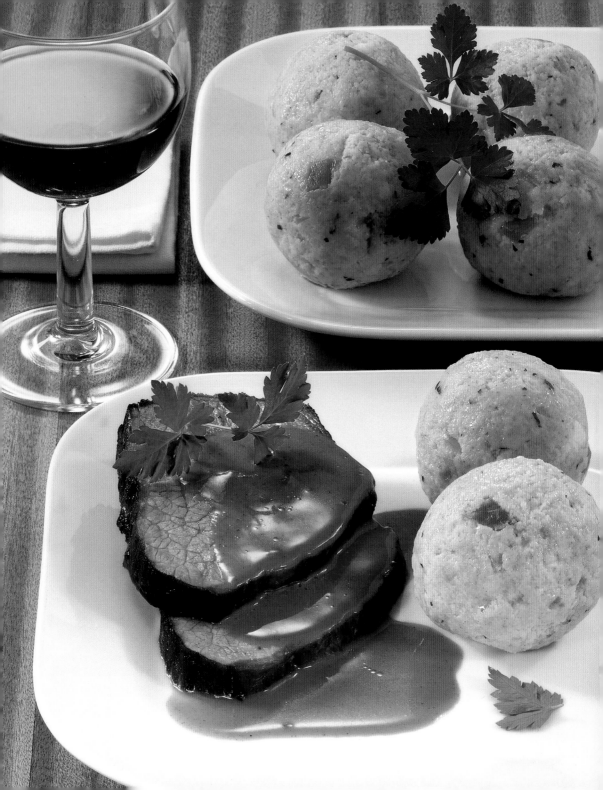

Pancake wraps with meat filling

SERVES 4

FOR THE BATTER

3 eggs

200 g (6½ oz) gluten-free
   plain flour

200 ml (7 fl oz/¾ cup) milk

1 tbsp oil

200 ml (7 fl oz/¾ cup) cold water

1 generous pinch salt

FOR THE FILLING

1 onion

2 garlic cloves

6 tbsp oil

400 g (13 oz) lean minced beef

2 tbsp tomato paste (purée)

salt, pepper, nutmeg

100 ml (3 fl oz/½ cup) red wine (or
   vegetable stock)

1-2 tsp cornflour (cornstarch)

4 tbsp cream

1 tsp dried herbs
   (e.g. herbes de Provence)

PREPARATION about 40 mins

1. Stir the eggs, then whisk in the flour, milk, oil, water and salt. Leave the batter to rise for about 20 minutes. Add a little more water if needed.

2. To make the filling, peel and finely dice the onion and garlic. In a frying pan, heat 2 tablespoons oil, add onion and garlic and sauté until translucent. Add the minced beef and fry until it becomes crumbly.

3. Stir in the tomato paste, then season with salt, pepper and nutmeg and fry for 3 more minutes, stirring constantly. Pour in the wine. Dissolve the cornflour in a little water, then stir into the mixture to thicken. Stir in the cream and the herbs.

4. Preheat the oven to 50°C (120°F). Heat the oil in a nonstick pan, and cook the pancakes, one after the other. Spread with the meat filling, then roll up and keep warm in the oven until ready to serve. Tastes great with a crispy green salad.

TIP

If you have some pancake batter left over, add a little more liquid and cook some thin pancakes. Cut the pancakes into thin strips and serve in a homemade soup.
This would be delicious, for example, with a Chinese chicken soup or with an old-fashioned beef broth.

VARIATION

Preheat the oven to 200°C (390°F)/180°C (355°F) fan-forced (middle shelf). Place the filled pancakes into a baking dish, then sprinkle 50 g (1⅔ oz) grated cheese over the top. Bake for about 20 minutes.

NUTRITIONAL VALUES PER PORTION:
670 Cal • 31 g protein • 38 g fat • 48 g carbohydrate

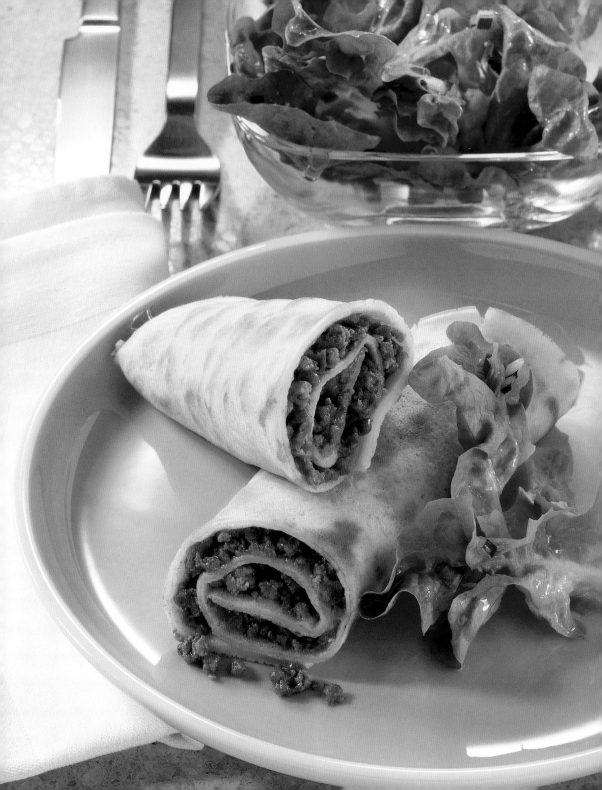

Burritos with chicken filling

SERVES 2

MAKES 4 BURRITOS

120 g (4 oz) maize flour

120 g (4 oz) gluten-free plain flour

1 pinch salt

2 tbsp oil

300 ml (10 fl oz/1¼ cup) water

2 tbsp oil

FOR THE FILLING

250 g (8 oz) chicken breast fillets

1 onion

1-2 garlic cloves

2 tbsp oil

400 g (13 oz) tinned chopped
      tomatoes

1 tbsp sweet paprika

1 tsp hot paprika

salt

1 pinch chilli powder

1 pinch sugar

2 tbsp oil

PREPARATION about 50 mins

1. To make the burritos put both kinds of flour into a bowl, add the salt, oil and water, then stir until you have a smooth batter. Add more water if needed. Leave to rise for 20 minutes.

2. To make the filling, wash the meat, pat it dry, then cut it into small dice. Peel and finely chop the onion and the garlic. Heat the oil in a frying pan, add the chicken dice and fry briefly. Add the onion and the garlic and continue frying.

3. Pour in the chopped tomatoes with their juice and season with salt and the two types of paprika. Continue cooking the filling until it has thickened a little, then season with chilli powder and sugar.

4. Preheat the oven to 50°C (120°F). Heat the oil in a nonstick frying pan. Add 3–4 tablespoons dough at a time to the frying pan, smooth it with the back of a moistened spoon and fry on both sides until crisp. Cover the burritos with aluminium foil and put them in the oven to keep warm. Place the hot filling on top of the burritos and fold them over or roll them up. Serve immediately with a green salad if desired.

VARIATION

Preheat the oven to 200°C (390°F)/180°C (355°F) fan-forced (middle shelf). Sprinkle the burritos with 50 g (1⅔ oz) grated cheese and bake them for 8-10 minutes in the oven until the cheese has melted. If you like vegetables, replace the meat with 300 g (10 oz) vegetables, for example capsicum (pepper) or zucchini (courgette).

TIP

If you're in a hurry you could just use a ready-made gluten-free salsa as a sauce with the fried chicken breasts instead of making one from scratch.

NUTRITIONAL VALUES PER PORTION:

427 Cal • 19 g protein • 17 g fat • 48 g carbohydrate

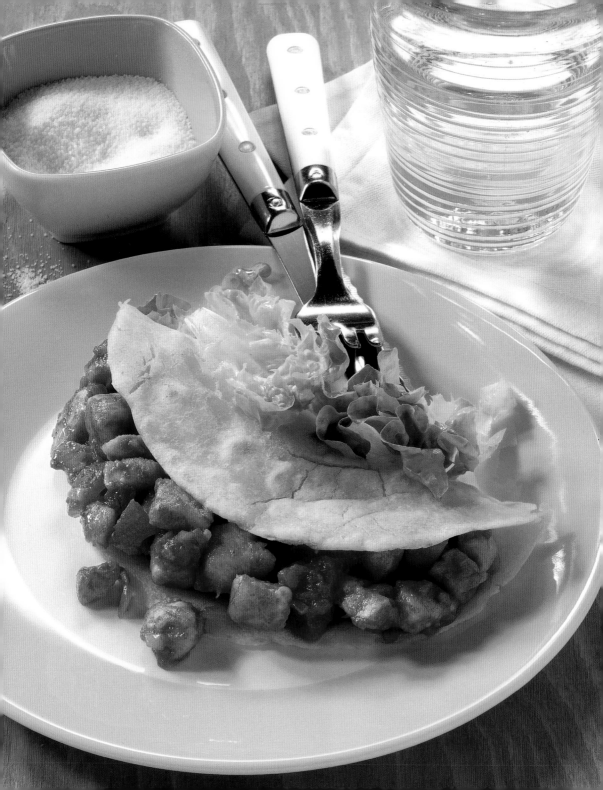

Zucchini Tortilla

SERVES 4

300 g (10 oz) zucchini (courgette)

2 small onions

2 garlic cloves

50 g (1²/₃ oz) salami or ham

6 tbsp olive oil

6 eggs

salt, pepper

1 tbsp chopped oregano

PREPARATION about 30 mins

1. Wash the zucchini, then cut them into small dice. Peel and finely chop the onions and the garlic. Cut the salami into small dice. In a frying pan, heat 2 tablespoons olive oil, add the onion and garlic and fry until translucent. Add the salami and zucchini dice and fry over medium heat for about 5 minutes.

2. In a large bowl, whisk the eggs, season with salt and pepper. Add the zucchini mixture to the eggs and stir in the chopped oregano. Heat 2 tablespoons oil in the frying pan. Pour in the zucchini and egg mixture and cook until the eggs set over low heat for about 5 minutes.

3. Let the tortilla slide onto a plate to turn it. Heat the remaining oil and fry the tortilla on the other side until a golden yellow. Serve immediately. This is tasty with a baguette or small potatoes fried in olive oil.

TIPS

This zucchini tortilla is equally tasty as a cold starter when served with the Spicy Barbecue Sauce on page 29.
For a slightly different version you can also replace the zucchini with the same amount of chopped leeks.

VARIATION

To make a potato tortilla, use 300 g (10 oz) cooked potato dice and 2 diced tomatoes instead of the zucchini.

NUTRITIONAL VALUES PER PORTION:
315 Cal • 13 g protein • 28 g fat • 2 g carbohydrate

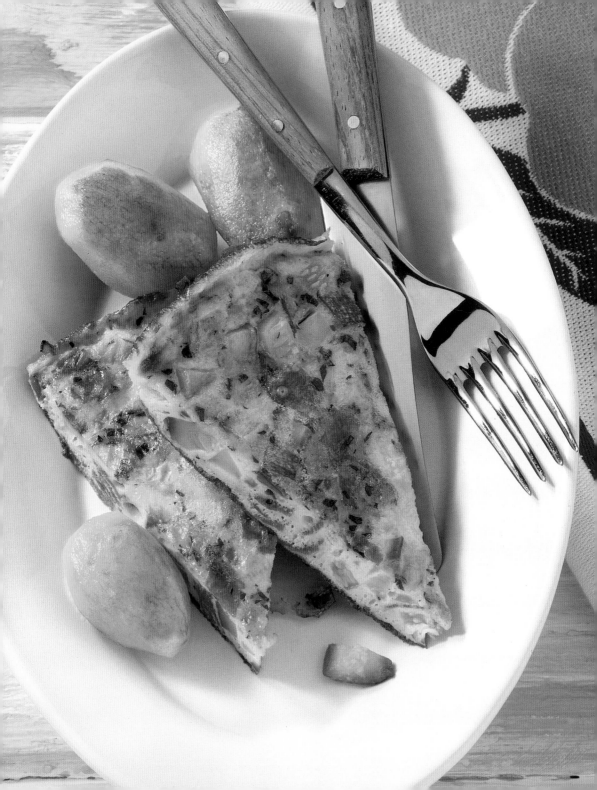

Basic recipe Pizza Dough

500 g (1 lb) gluten-free plain flour
1½ tsp dried yeast
1 tsp sea salt
1 tsp raw sugar
2 tbsp olive oil
450 ml (15 fl oz/1¾ cups)
  lukewarm water
PREPARATION about 20 mins
RISING about 30 mins

1. Combine the flour with the dried yeast, salt and sugar. Add oil and water and knead until you have a smooth dough.

2. Line the baking tray with baking paper. Roll out the dough, place it on the tray and place in a warm oven to rise for about 20 minutes (see Tip).

3. Cover the pizza with the topping of your choice (see page 50).

TIP

Gluten-free dough requires plenty of moisture in order to rise well. The following method has proved successful. Briefly preheat the oven to 50°C (120°F) , then turn it off (about 35°C/95°F). Place the rolled-out dough on the tray in the oven, then place a rack covered with a damp kitchen cloth on top. Before baking the pizza, make absolutely sure you remove the kitchen cloth first!

NUTRITIONAL VALUE:

1975 Cal • 15 g protein • 25 g fat • 427 g carbohydrate

Focaccia

**MAKES 2 X 8 PIECES
(2 ROUND TRAYS
30 CM/12 IN DIAMETER)**
butter for greasing
1 basic recipe Pizza Dough
  (see above)
100 ml (3 fl oz/½ cup) olive oil
4-5 tbsp fresh rosemary
PREPARATION about 20 mins
RISING about 20 mins
BAKING about 2 x 25 mins

1. Preheat the oven to 50°C (120°F), then turn it off. Grease the trays. Prepare the pizza dough, following the recipe. Roll out the dough, place it on the trays and place the trays in the warm oven to rise for 20 minutes (see Tip above).

2. Take the trays out of the oven. Preheat the oven to 250°C (480°F)/220°C (430°F) fan-forced (middle shelf). Heat the oil in a frying pan, add the rosemary, turn off the heat and leave to cook for 10 minutes.

3. Cut the dough crossways and brush with half the warm oil. Bake the breads in the preheated oven, one after the other (fan-forced both together, using the middle and the lower shelf), for 20–25 minutes.

4. Brush the hot breads with the remaining oil and serve hot. Focaccia are delicious when served with antipasti.

VARIATION

Instead of using rosemary you could try 2 crushed garlic cloves and 2-3 tablespoons dried Italian herbs and fry these in the oil. Then brush the hot focaccia with this oil as per the recipe.

NUTRITIONAL VALUES PER PORTION:

165 kcal • 1 g protein • 6 g fat • 26 g carbohydrate

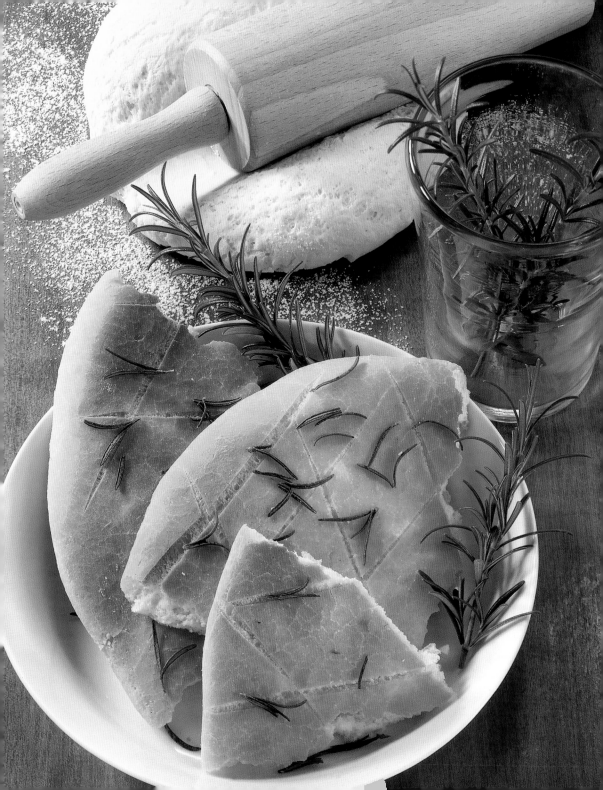

Colourful Family Pizza

**MAKES 16 SLICES
(1 BAKING TRAY OR
2 ROUND BAKING DISHES
28 CM/11 IN DIAMETER)**

800 g (1 lb 10 oz) tinned
   chopped tomatoes

1 basic recipe Pizza Dough
   (see page 48)

½ tsp salt

250 g (8 oz) mozzarella

1 tbsp dried Italian herbs
   (e.g. thyme, oregano)

2 tbsp olive oil

PREPARATION about 40 mins

RISING about 20 mins

BAKING about 25 mins

1. Preheat the oven to 250°C (480°F)/220°C (430°F) fan-forced (middle shelf). Drain the chopped tomatoes and cover the dough evenly with the tomato pieces; season with salt. Cut the mozzarella into small pieces and distribute evenly over the tomatoes.

2. Sprinkle the pizza with the herbs. Drizzle with olive oil and bake in the oven for about 20–25 minutes.

TIP

Catch the juice when you drain the chopped tomatoes and use it as a starting point for making a homemade tomato-based pasta sauce.

VARIATIONS

To make an Hawaiian pizza prepare a topping using 100 g (3⅓ oz) ham, cut into thin strips, and 5 slices of pineapple.

For a savoury alternative, use 100 g (3⅓ oz) salami, cut into strips, fresh button mushrooms slices and artichoke bottoms from the jar.

If you like fish, cover your pizza with tinned tuna. Add a few olives too – choose pitted ones that are marinated in oil.

For a sweet variation replace the olive oil with rapeseed oil, then spread the dough on the baking tray with 500 g (1 lb) mixed puréed berries. Slice 1 ball buffalo mozzarella and place on your sweet pizza. Just before baking, sprinkle with 2-3 tablespoons sugar.

NUTRITIONAL VALUES PER PORTION:
180 Cal • 5 g protein • 6 g fat • 28 g carbohydrate

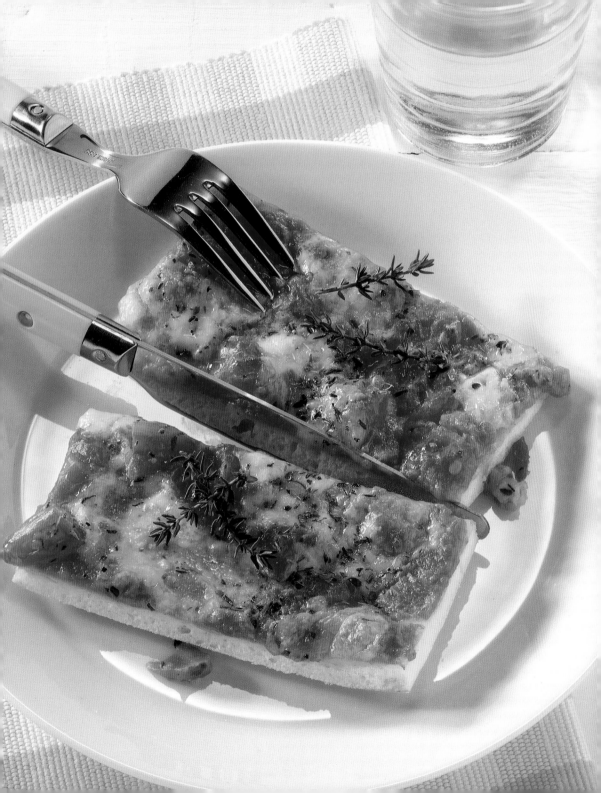

Polenta Pizza

**MAKES 16 SLICES
(1 BAKING TRAY)**
FOR THE DOUGH
750 ml (24 fl oz/3 cups) water
½ tsp salt
1 tbsp butter
250 g (8 oz) polenta
FOR THE TOPPING
800 g (1 lb 10 oz) tinned
  chopped tomatoes
125 g (4 oz) mozzarella
100 g (3⅓ oz) ham
salt, pepper
1 tbsp dried Italian herbs
1 tbsp olive oil
PREPARATION about 35 mins
RISING about 30 mins
BAKING about 25 mins

1. In a saucepan, bring the water together with the salt and the butter to the boil. Sprinkle in the polenta, cook for 5 minutes while stirring, then leave to swell for 30 minutes over the lowest temperature, stirring frequently.

2. Preheat the oven to 200°C (390°F)/180°C (355°F) fan-forced (middle shelf). Line the baking tray with baking paper. Tip the tomatoes into a sieve and leave to drain. Spread the polenta about 2 cm (¾ in) thick onto the prepared tray. This will not cover the tray entirely. Leave to cool.

3. Cover the polenta with the drained tomato pieces. Cut the mozzarella into pieces and the ham into strips, then distribute both evenly on the pizza. Season with salt and pepper. Sprinkle the dried herbs on top. Drizzle the olive oil on top.

4. Bake in the oven for about 25 minutes. Serve hot. This goes well with a mixed salad.

TIP

You can use any topping of your choice: for example, instead of the ham, use salami or tinned tuna.

VARIATION

Polenta is equally delicious served as open sandwiches!
To make these, prepare the polenta as in Step 1 and spread it 2 cm (¾ in) thick onto a tray lined with baking paper. Leave to cool. Whisk 2 eggs in a deep plate. Grate 100 g (3⅓ oz) Parmesan and combine with 2 tablespoons gluten-free breadcrumbs on a second plate. Once it has cooled down, cut the polenta slab into squares or rectangles. Turn the polenta slices first in the whisked eggs, then in the grated cheese and breadcrumb mixture. In a frying pan, heat 3 tablespoons oil. Add the slices and fry them on both sides until they are golden brown.

NUTRITIONAL VALUES PER PORTION:
98 Cal • 5 g protein • 3 g fat • 13 g carbohydrate

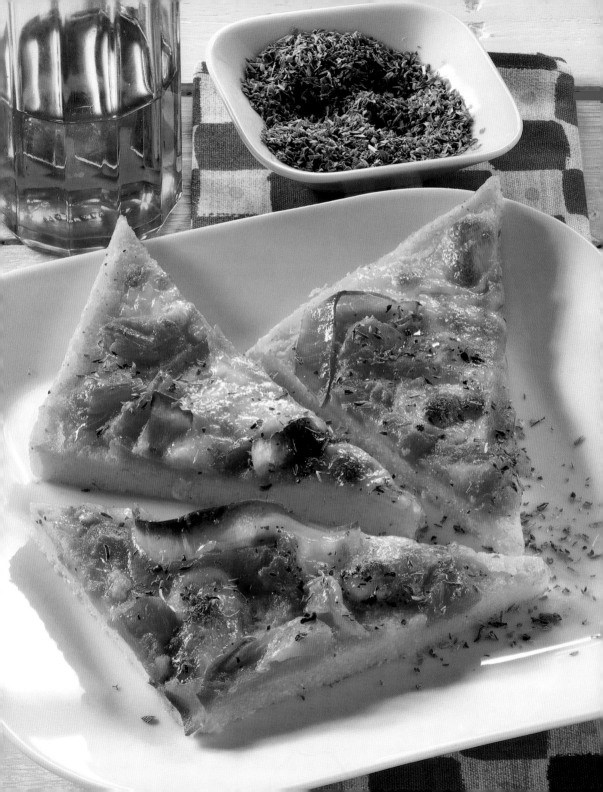

Basic recipe Yeast Dough

**MAKES 16 SLICES
(1 BAKING TRAY)**

butter for greasing

250 g (8 oz) gluten-free plain flour

1½ tsp dried yeast

125 g (4 oz) low-fat cream cheese

60 ml (2 fl oz/¼ cup) oil

½ tsp salt

1 egg

PREPARATION about 15 mins

RISING about 20 mins

1. Grease the baking tray. Combine the flour with the dried yeast. Thoroughly knead in the cream cheese, oil, salt and egg. (Add a little more water, if needed.) Roll out the dough, place it on the baking tray and place in a warm oven for about 20 minutes to rise (see Tip on page 48).

2. Cover the yeast pastry with the topping of your choice (for example, see recipe below).

VARIATION

This dough is an excellent basis for fruit cakes and crumbles. Simply add only a pinch salt instead of the ½ teaspoon used here, but add 50 g (1²⁄₃ oz) sugar and a pinch grated lemon zest. Before baking, cover with the fruit topping of your choice.

NUTRITIONAL VALUES PER PORTION:

90 Cal • 2 g protein • 3 g fat • 14 g carbohydrate

French Onion Tart

**MAKES 20 SLICES
(1 BAKING TRAY)**

butter for greasing

1 basic recipe Yeast Dough
   (see above)

1 kg (2 lb 4 oz) onions

2 tbsp oil

125 g (4 oz) sour cream

3 eggs

2 tbsp gluten-free plain flour

salt, pepper

50 g (1²⁄₃ oz) bacon dice

caraway seeds (if desired)

PREPARATION about 1 hr

RISING about 20 mins

BAKING about 40 mins

1. Prepare the yeast dough to the recipe above. Grease the baking tray. Roll out the dough and place it on the tray, forming an edge of about 2 cm (¾ in). Place the tray in a warm oven and allow to rise for about 20 minutes (see Tip on page 48).

2. Meanwhile, peel and roughly dice the onions. In a frying pan, heat the oil and fry the onion until translucent. Leave the onion mixture to cool a little, then combine it with the sour cream, the eggs and the flour. Season with salt and pepper. Remove the tray from the oven.

3. Preheat the oven to 220°C (430°F)/200°C (390°F) fan-forced (middle shelf). Spread the onion mixture on the dough, then spread the bacon dice on top and sprinkle on a few caraway seeds, if desired. Bake the onion tart for 30–40 minutes until golden. Cut the tart into rectangular pieces and serve hot.

TIP

Once baked and cooled down, the onion tart can easily be frozen; it will taste just as delicious when warmed up!

NUTRITIONAL VALUES PER PORTION:

150 Cal • 3 g protein • 7 g fat • 17 g carbohydrate

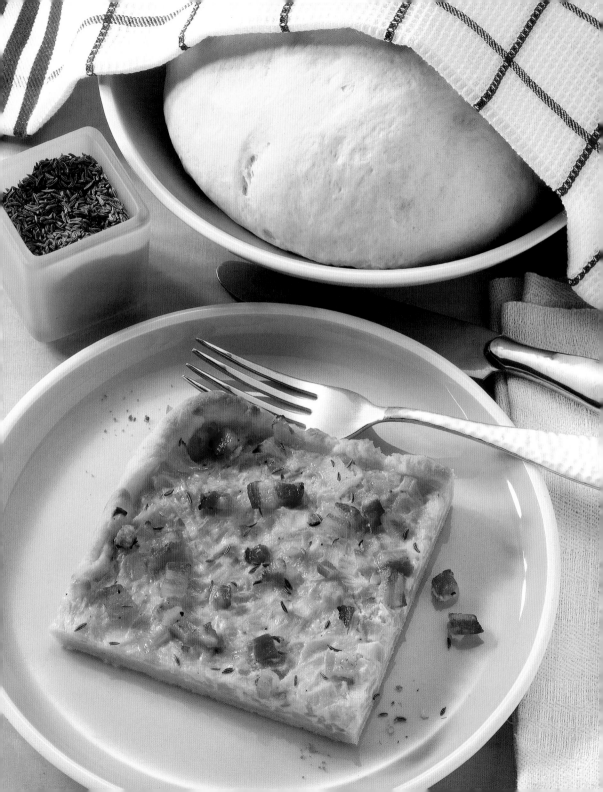

Basic recipe Cream Cheese and Oil Pastry

150 g (5 oz) low-fat cream cheese
6 tbsp milk
6 tbsp rapeseed oil
1 pinch salt
300 g (10 oz) gluten-free plain flour
1 tbsp cream of tartar
flour, for dusting
PREPARATION about 15 mins

1. Stir the cream cheese with the milk, oil and salt until well combined. Combine the flour with the baking powder and add. Knead all the ingredients to make a dough. Add a little more flour if needed.

2. Carefully roll out the dough and continue working according to the recipe (see page 58).

TIP
This dough is a good basis for sweet as well as baked goods. You'll find some delicious recipes for using this cream cheese and oil dough on page 58.

NUTRITIONAL VALUE:
1745 Cal • 29 g protein • 66 g fat • 259 g carbohydrate

Basic recipe Cream Cheese Puff Pastry

250 g (8 oz) gluten-free plain flour
2 tbsp baking powder
1 pinch salt
200 g (6½ oz) low-fat cream cheese
160 g (5⅓ oz) margarine
flour, for dusting
PREPARATION about 30 mins
RISING about 30 mins

1. Combine the flour with the baking powder and the salt. Lightly squeeze out the cream cheese in a kitchen cloth, then add to the flour together with the margarine. Knead until you have a smooth dough.

2. Dust the work surface with flour, then roll out the dough, about 1–2 cm (½–¾ in) thick, to make a square. Fold the dough sheet in towards the middle from the left and the right as well as from the top and the bottom. Roll it out again, then repeat the turning in process, always sprinkling a little flour onto the dough while doing so.

3. Wrap the dough in cling film and chill in the refrigerator for 30 minutes. Roll out and continue working to the recipe (see page 58).

TIP
This dough is excellent for baking both sweet and savoury foods. You can find delicious savoury and sweet recipes for this Cream Cheese Puff Pastry on page 58.

NUTRITIONAL VALUE:
2160 Cal • 33 g protein • 132 g fat • 217 g carbohydrate

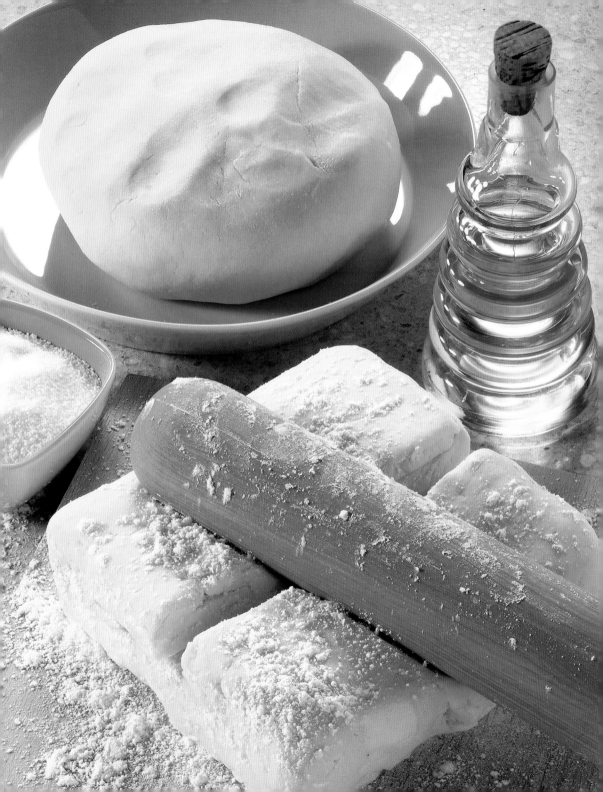

Meat Parcels

MAKES 20

1 basic recipe Cream Cheese and
   Oil Pastry or 1 basic recipe
   Cream Cheese Puff Pastry
   (see page 56)

1 onion

½ bunch parsley

2 tbsp oil

1 small red capsicum (pepper)

50 g (1²/₃ oz) hard cheese
   (e.g. Emmental)

400 g (13 oz) minced beef

2 eggs

2 tbsp gluten-free breadcrumbs

salt, pepper

1 tbsp milk

flour, for dusting

PREPARATION about 20 mins

BAKING about 25 mins

1. Preheat the oven to 220°C (430°F)/200°C (390°F) fan-forced (middle shelf). Line two baking trays with baking paper. Prepare the dough according to one of the basic recipes. Dust the work surface, then roll out the dough to about 3 mm. Cut into squares of about 10–12 cm (4–5 in).

2. Peel and finely chop the onion. Wash and finely chop the parsley. Heat 2 tablespoons oil in a nonstick pan, then sauté the onion dice until translucent. Add the parsley and fry it. Leave to cool.

3. Wash the capsicum, trim, then finely dice it. Dice the cheese. Place both in a large bowl together with the onion and herb mixture and the minced beef. Add 1 egg and the breadcrumbs and thoroughly combine. Season with salt and pepper.

4. Place 1 tablespoon of the minced beef mixture on each of the dough squares. Separate the second egg. Brush the dough edges with the egg white, fold them diagonally across and press together with a fork.

5. Stir together the egg yolk and the milk, then brush the pastry triangles with the mixture. Bake the parcels in the oven for about 20–25 minutes until golden. Leave to cool on a rack.

SWEET VARIATIONS

To make apple turnovers, core and chop 4–5 apples. Briefly bring to the boil water, a little sugar and the apple. Drain, catching the water, and use this to soak 4 tablespoons raisins. Leave the apples to cool a little, then combine with the raisins, 2 tablespoons chopped almonds and a pinch cinnamon. Spoon the mix onto the dough squares. Turn the corners of the squares towards the middle, press the edges together and continue as for the meat parcels.
To make nut croissants, combine 250 g (8 oz) chopped hazelnuts and 4½ tablespoons sugar, a few drops vanilla essence and 100 g (3⅓ oz) cream until you have a pulpy mix. Place 1 tablespoon mixture on each square. Roll up from the corner, shape as croissants and continue as for the meat parcels.

SAVOURY VARIATION

To make prosciutto croissants replace the minced beef with 150 g (5 oz) ham and 100 g (3⅓ oz) prosciutto. Finely chop both meats, then place 1 tablespoon of the mixed dice in the middle of each dough square. Roll the parcel up from one of the corners, squeezing the sides together, then continue as in the Meat Parcel recipe on this page.

NUTRITIONAL VALUES PER PORTION:
163 Cal • 7 g protein • 9 g fat • 14 g carbohydrate

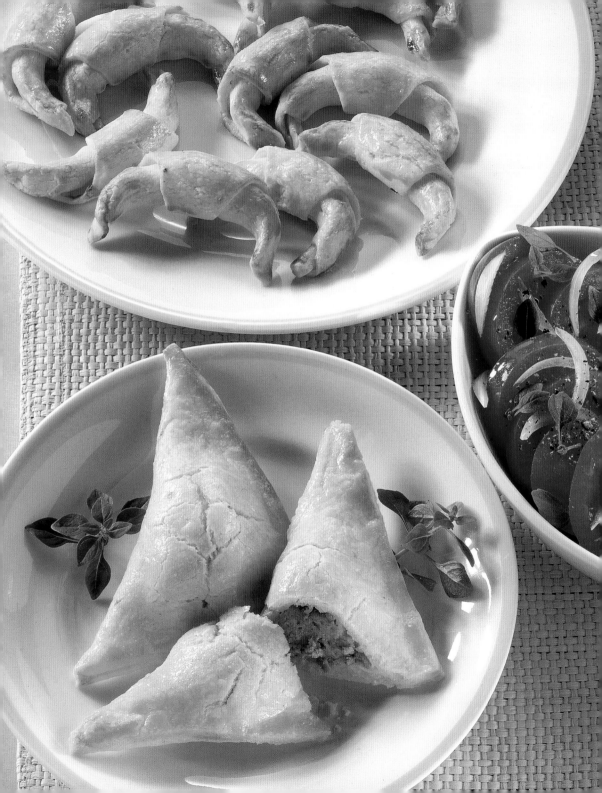

Leek Quiche

**MAKES 12 SLICES
(1 LOOSE-BOTTOMED TIN
28 CM/11 IN DIAMETER)**

FOR THE DOUGH

220 g (7 oz) gluten-free plain flour

100 g (3⅓ oz) cold butter

1 generous pinch salt

3 tbsp cold water

FOR THE TOPPING

300 g (10 oz) leek

2 tbsp olive oil

150 ml (5 fl oz/¾ cup) milk

100 g (3⅓ oz) cream

3 eggs

salt, pepper

50 g (1⅔ oz) grated Emmental

butter for greasing

PREPARATION about 40 mins

CHILLING about 1 hr

BAKING about 40 mins

1. Knead a dough from the flour, butter, salt and water. Add more water or flour if needed. Wrap the dough in cling film and place in the refrigerator to chill for about 1 hour.

2. Preheat the oven to 200°C (390°F)/180°C (355°F) fan-forced (middle shelf). Line the tin with baking paper and lightly grease. Roll out the dough and place it in the tin, shaping an edge of about 2 cm (¾ in).

3. Trim and thoroughly wash the leeks, then cut them into strips about 1 cm (½ in) thick. Heat the oil in a frying pan, add the leek strips and sauté them for about 5 minutes.

4. Whisk the milk with the cream and the eggs. Season with salt and pepper. Stir in the leeks and the cheese. Spread the mixture over the dough, and bake the quiche in the oven for about 30–40 minutes. Serve while still hot.

TIP

Add some small bacon dice when frying the leeks.

VARIATION

To make a zucchini quiche, you will need:

300 g (10 oz) zucchini
   (courgette)

2 tbsp olive oil

1 garlic clove

200 g (6½ oz) cream

2 eggs

salt, pepper

Wash and trim, then slice the zucchini. Heat the oil in a frying pan and sauté the zucchini for about 3 minutes. Leave to cool a little, then finely chop. Whisk the cream with the eggs and the garlic. Season to taste with salt and pepper. Stir the zucchini slices into the mixture and spread evenly on top of the dough. Bake as for the Leek Quiche in the recipe.

NUTRITIONAL VALUES PER PORTION:
220 Cal • 4 g protein • 15 g fat • 17 g carbohydrate

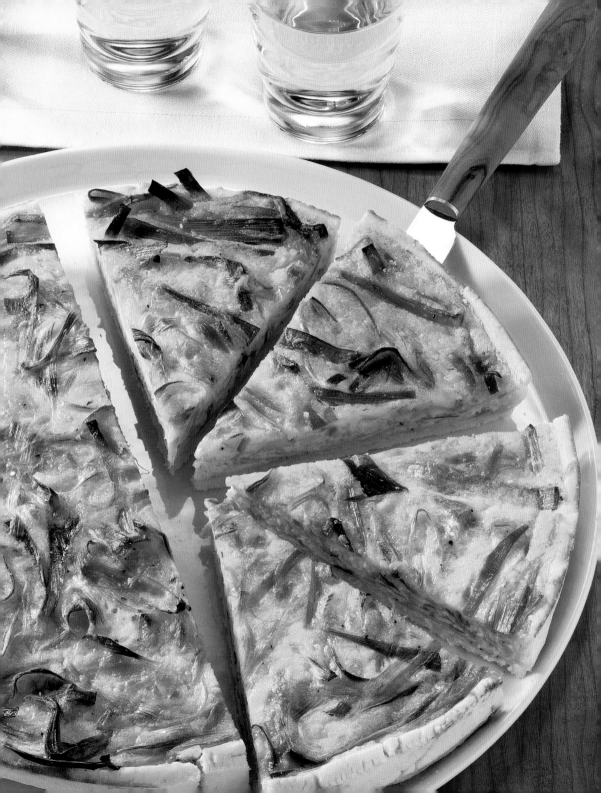

Cheese Bites

MAKES 2 X 10 SLICES (2 BAKING TRAYS)

FOR THE DOUGH

150 g (5 oz) finely ground amaranth (from the health food store, or buckwheat)

150 g (5 oz) gluten-free plain flour

2 tsp guar gum (from the health food store)

1 tsp cream of tartar

120 g (4 oz) cold butter

100 g (3⅓ oz) low-fat cream cheese

1 tsp salt

1 egg

100 g (3⅓ oz) grated strong hard cheese

1 egg yolk

1 tbsp milk

FOR SPRINKLING

caraway seeds, shelled sesame seeds, poppy seeds, coarse sea salt, chopped pistachios or almonds

PREPARATION about 25 mins

CHILLING about 1 hr

BAKING about 2 x15 mins

1. Combine the ground amaranth with the other two types of flour and the cream of tartar; put onto a baking board or in a large bowl. Add the butter cut into small pats. Stir together the cream cheese with the salt, egg and grated cheese. Knead with the flour mixture to form a smooth dough. Wrap the dough in cling film and chill for 1 hour.

2. Preheat the oven to 220°C (430°F)/200°C (390°F) fan-forced (middle shelf). Line the baking trays with baking paper. On a flour-dusted surface, roll out the dough to a rectangle about 6 mm (¼ in) thick. With a knife or a pie crimper, cut diamond shapes of about 3 cm by 6 cm (1¼ by 2⅓ in). Place the diamonds on the trays.

3. Whisk the egg yolk with the milk, then use to brush the pastry. Sprinkle with your choice of topping – caraway seeds, sesame seeds, poppy seeds, coarse sea salt, chopped pistachios or almonds. Bake the cheese bites in batches for 12–15 minutes until golden. Place on a rack to cool.

TIPS

Why not use some cookie cutters for a change? These cheese bites are just as attractive when shaped as hearts, stars or rings.

The cheese bites will keep well if stored in a biscuit tin, for about one week – unless they are eaten sooner!

NUTRITIONAL VALUES PER PORTION:
150 Cal • 5 g protein • 9 g fat • 12 g carbohydrate

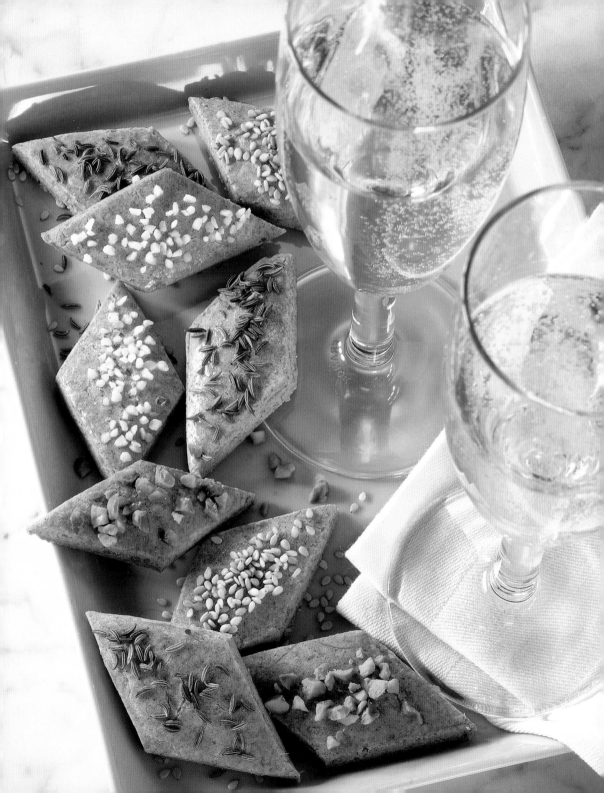

French Apple Crumble

SERVES 6

butter for greasing

4-6 apples (e.g. Golden Delicious or Granny Smith)

3-4 tbsp sugar

100-125 g (3⅓-4 oz) gluten-free plain flour

50 g (1⅔ oz) ground almonds

100 g (3⅓ oz) sugar

½ tsp cinnamon

75 g (2¾ oz) butter

PREPARATION about 30 mins
BAKING about 30 mins

1. Preheat the oven to 200°C (390°F)/175°C (345°F) fan-forced (middle shelf). Grease an ovenproof dish. Peel the apples and cut them into wedges. Bring to the boil in a little water together with the sugar. (The apples should still be firm to the bite.) Tip into a sieve and drain, then place in the dish.

2. To make the crumble, combine the flour with the almonds, sugar and cinnamon. Add the butter as small pats and work into crumble. Add more flour or butter if needed.

3. Sprinkle the crumble over the apples. Bake in the oven for about 25–30 minutes, or until the crumble is lightly browned. Serve the crumble hot.

VARIATION

Try using mixed berries instead of apples. These will not need to be cooked first. You can replace the cinnamon with a few drops of vanilla essence. The baking time is the same.

NUTRITIONAL VALUES PER PORTION:
270 Cal • 2 g protein • 16 g fat • 28 g carbohydrate

Red Jelly with custard

SERVES 4
FOR THE RED JELLY

500 g (1 lb) red summer fruit (e.g. strawberries, redcurrants, raspberries and cherries)

2 tbsp sugar

3 tbsp cornflour (cornstarch)

FOR THE CUSTARD

250 ml (8 fl oz/1 cup) + 3 tbsp milk

1-2 tbsp sugar

a few drops vanilla essence

1 heaped tsp cornflour (cornstarch)

1 egg yolk

2 tbsp cream

PREPARATION about 30 mins
CHILLING about 2 hrs

1. To make the red jelly, clean the fruit, hull and halve the strawberries, stone the cherries and bring to the boil together with the sugar. Cook for 2 minutes. Dissolve the cornflour in 3 tablespoons cold water, add the mixture to the fruits and bring to the boil. Cook for a further 2 minutes. Fill the mixture into a bowl, cover and chill for 2 hours.

2. To make the vanilla custard, bring 250 ml (8 fl oz/1 cup) milk to the boil together with the sugar and the vanilla essence. Dissolve the cornflour in 3 tablespoons cold milk, then stir into the bubbling liquid. Bring back the mixture to the boil, remove from the heat.

3. Whisk together the egg yolk and the cream, then stir into the hot liquid; do not allow to boil again. Leave the sauce to cool. Frequently stir the custard so that no skin starts to form. Serve the red jelly with the custard.

TIP

Instead of fresh fruit you can just as easily use a pack of frozen mixed berries.

NUTRITIONAL VALUES PER PORTION:
235 Cal • 4 g protein • 7 g fat • 37 g carbohydrate

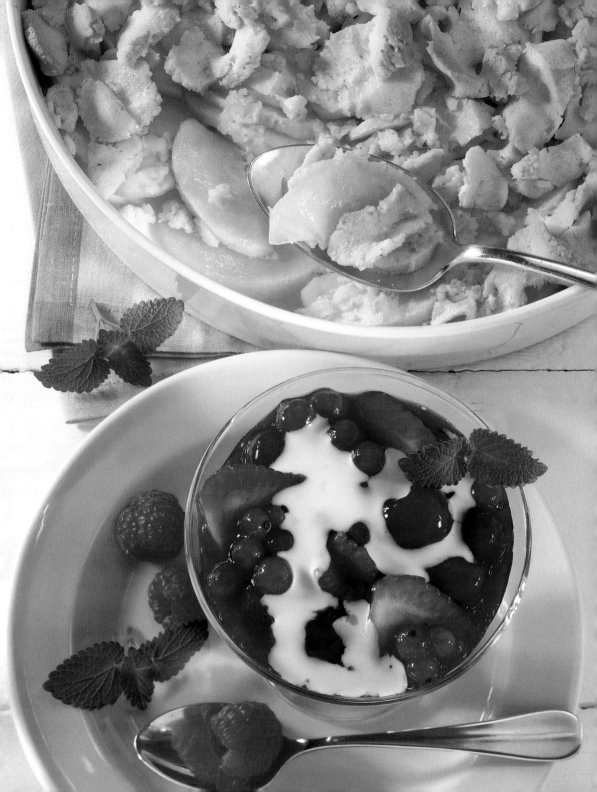

Light Orange Mousse

SERVES 4-6

70 g (2½ oz) powdered gelatine

300 ml (10 fl oz/1¼ cups) freshly
squeezed orange juice

2 eggs

80 g (2¾ oz) sugar

3 tbsp orange liqueur (if liked)

200 g (6½ oz) cream

1 untreated orange

> **VARIATION**
>
> If you are making the dessert
> around the festive season, simply
> add a pinch each cinnamon and
> ground cloves.

PREPARATION about 40 mins

CHILLING about 4 hrs

1. Soak the gelatine and leave to swell according to packet instructions.

2. Warm the orange juice, then stir in the gelatine until dissolved. Leave the mixture to cool.

3. Separate the eggs. Beat the egg yolks with the sugar until foamy. Stir into the orange jelly, then add the liqueur.

4. Beat the cream until stiff and beat the egg whites until they stand in stiff peaks. Fold both into the cold mixture. Cover and chill for about 4 hours.

5. Wash and brush the orange under hot water, then pat dry. Thinly grate the zest, and peel the orange. Using two tablespoons, cut off shapes from the orange mousse and place on a plate. Garnish with orange segments and sprinkle with the zest.

NUTRITIONAL VALUES PER PORTION:

275 Cal • 6 g protein • 15 g fat • 24 g carbohydrate

Scandinavian Buttermilk Cream

SERVES 4-6

70 g (2½ oz) powdered gelatine

500 ml (16 fl oz/2 cups) buttermilk

4 tbsp sugar

a few drops vanilla essence

200 g (6½ oz) whipping cream

500 g (1 lb) strawberries

1 tsp sugar

50 g (1⅔ oz) flaked almonds

> **VARIATION**
>
> A cherry sauce also goes well with
> this dessert. Bring preserved sour
> cherries to the boil with a cinnamon
> stick and sugar. Thicken with 2
> teaspoons cornflour. Serve the
> sauce hot with the buttermilk cream.

PREPARATION about 30 mins

CHILLING about 4 hrs

1. Soak the gelatine and leave to swell according to packet instructions.

2. Stir the sugar and the vanilla essence into the buttermilk. Heat the gelatine in a saucepan without letting it boil. Stir the dissolved gelatine first into 2–3 tablespoons of the sugared buttermilk, then into the remaining buttermilk.

3. As soon as the buttermilk mixture starts to jellify, beat the cream until stiff. Fold the whipped cream into the buttermilk and leave to chill for 4 hours.

4. To make the fruit sauce, wash, drain and hull the strawberries, then purée them together with the sugar. Dry-roast the almonds in a frying pan without fat until you can smell them. Just before serving, sprinkle the buttermilk cream with the almonds and serve with the strawberry sauce.

NUTRITIONAL VALUES PER PORTION:

335 Cal • 9 g protein • 22 g fat • 27 g carbohydrate

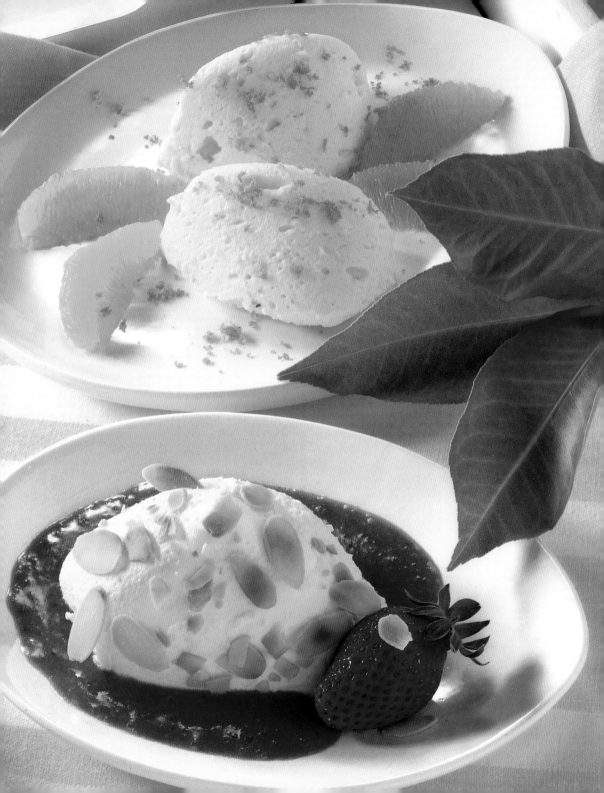

Belgian Waffles

MAKES 8 WAFFLES

125 g (4 oz) softened butter

3½ tbsp raw sugar

1 pinch salt

a few drops vanilla essence

3 eggs

200 g (6½ oz) buckwheat flour

50 g (1⅔ oz) potato or cornflour

2 level tsp baking powder

250 ml (8 fl oz/1 cup) milk

oil, for the waffle iron

icing sugar, for dusting

PREPARATION about 20 mins

BAKING about 8 x5 mins

1. Whisk the butter with the sugar, salt, vanilla essence and the eggs until very foamy. Combine the flour with the cornflour and the baking powder, then stir with the milk into the batter.

2. Brush the waffle iron with the oil and heat it. Place 1 small ladle of batter into the hot waffle iron at a time and bake for about 5 minutes until golden. Dust the waffles with icing sugar and serve immediately.

TIP

The waffles are ideal for a children's party. You can make them to order, for example with jam, nut or nougat spread, stewed apple, fresh strawberries or simply whipped cream.

VARIATIONS

Stir 1 tablespoon chopped almonds or hazelnuts into the batter. Or grate a fresh apple into the waffle batter for a deliciously fruity option.

NUTRITIONAL VALUES PER PORTION:

370 Cal • 6 g protein • 22 g fat • 38 g carbohydrate

German Cream Cheese Potato Cakes

SERVES 4

75 g (2¾ oz) raisins

500 g (1 lb) cooked floury potatoes
   (from the day before if possible)

2 eggs

250 g (8 oz) cream cheese

75 g (2¾ oz) sugar

1 pinch cinnamon

1 tsp grated zest
   of 1 untreated lemon

1 pinch salt

50 g (1⅔ oz) gluten-free
   plain flour

100 g (3⅓ oz) clarified butter
   for frying

cinnamon and sugar for sprinkling

PREPARATION about 45 mins

1. Soak the raisins in boiling water. Slip the skins off the cooked potatoes and push the potatoes through a ricer. Combine the eggs with the cream cheese, sugar, cinnamon, lemon zest and salt and add to the potatoes. Knead the flour and the raisins into the mixture.

2. Heat the clarified butter in a frying pan. Using a tablespoon, cut off small pats, place them into the frying pan and squash them flat. Fry the potato cakes until golden on both sides. Sprinkle with cinnamon and sugar and serve hot. The potato cakes are delicious with vanilla custard or stewed apples.

TIP

Keep the Potato Cakes warm in a preheated oven until you are ready to serve.

NUTRITIONAL VALUES PER PORTION:

585 Cal • 13 g protein • 26 g fat • 75 g carbohydrate

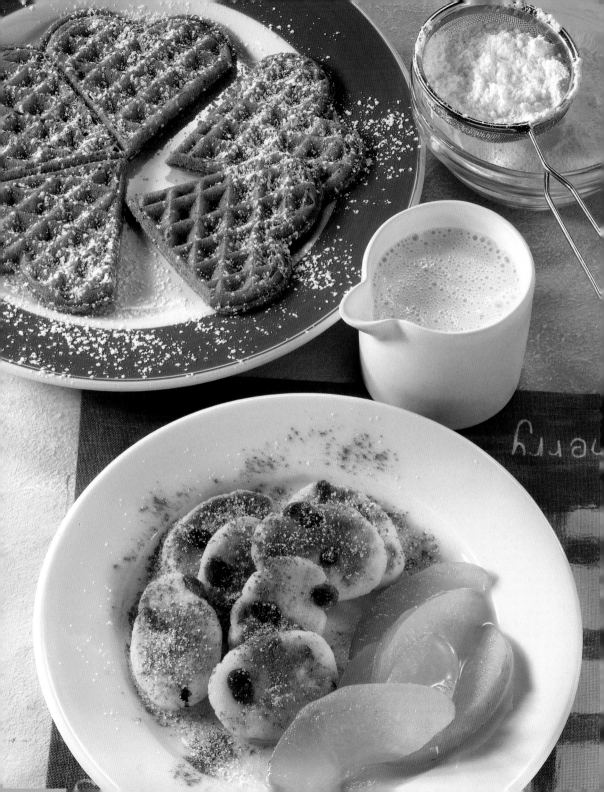

Rice and Cream Cheese Gratin with apples

SERVES 4

200 g (6½ oz) pudding rice

600 ml (20 fl oz/2½ cups) milk

1 pinch salt

2 eggs

7 tbsp sugar

250 g (8 oz) low-fat cream cheese

½ tsp grated zest
   of 1 untreated lemon

3 apples (e.g. Golden Delicious
   or Granny Smith)

3 tbsp flaked almonds

1 tbsp butter in small pats

butter for greasing

PREPARATION about 30 mins

BAKING about 40 mins

NUTRITIONAL VALUES PER PORTION:

580 Cal • 22 g protein • 16 g fat • 86 g carbohydrate

1. Wash the rice under cold water. Heat the milk, then add the rice and the salt. Leave the rice to simmer over a low temperature for about 15 minutes; do not allow it to get too soft.

2. Preheat the oven to 200°C (390°F)/180°C (355°F) fan-forced (middle shelf). Lightly grease the baking dish. Separate the eggs. Whisk the egg yolks with the sugar until foamy, then stir in the cream cheese and the lemon zest. Once the rice has cooled a little, combine it with the egg yolk mixture. Whisk the egg whites until stiff, then gently fold them into the mixture.

3. Pour half the mixture into the dish. Peel, core and thinly slice the apples, place on top of the mixture. Spread the remaining rice mixture on top. Sprinkle with flaked almonds and little pats of butter. Bake in the oven for about 40 minutes until golden. Serve with stewed fruit.

TIP

If you like them, soak 2 tablespoons sultanas in boiling water, then sprinkle them together with the apple slices over the rice mixture in the dish.

Sweet Millet Gratin

SERVES 4

400 g (13 oz) millet

400 ml (14 fl oz/1 ¾ cup) water

600 ml (20 fl oz/2½ cups) milk

butter for greasing

½ untreated lemon

80 g (2¾ oz) sultanas

1-2 tbsp honey

½ tsp cardamom

½ tsp cinnamon

1½ tsp sugar

a few drops vanilla essence

50 g (1⅔ oz) hazelnut kernels

1 tbsp butter in small pats

PREPARATION about 30 mins

BAKING about 30 mins

NUTRITIONAL VALUES PER PORTION:

495 Cal • 14 g protein • 16 g fat • 76 g carbohydrate

1. In a saucepan, bring the millet to the boil with the water and the milk, then leave to simmer for 15–20 minutes.

2. Preheat the oven to 200°C (390°F)/180°C (355°F) fan-forced (middle shelf). Grease the baking dish. Wash the lemon under hot water, pat dry. Thinly grate the zest, squeeze out the juice. Stir into the hot millet together with the raisins, honey, cardamom, cinnamon, sugar and vanilla essence.

3. Pour the mixture into the dish. Chop the hazelnuts and sprinkle them on top, then set the butter pats on top. Bake in the oven for about 25–30 minutes until golden. Serve hot. Delicious with stewed plums or apples!

VARIATIONS

Add some fresh fruit, such as apple or pear slices, to the millet mixture before baking.

As a tasty variation on the raisins you can also use cranberries or chopped almonds for a taste variation.

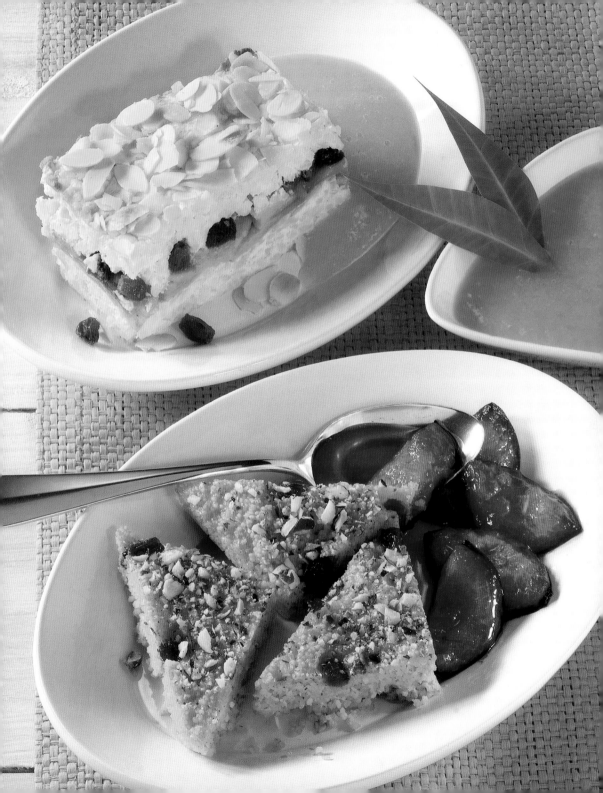

Raspberry Tiramisu

SERVES 6

1 basic recipe Almond Sponge
   (see below, variation)
40 ml (1⅓ fl oz) raspberry
   schnapps (if desired)
300 g (10 oz) raspberries
500 g (1 lb) low-fat cream cheese
250 g (8 oz) mascarpone
155 g (5 oz) sugar
a few drops vanilla essence
200 g (6½ oz) cream

PREPARATION about 40 mins
BAKING about 30 mins
CHILLING about 4 hrs

1. Prepare the almond sponge according to the basic recipe (see below). Leave to cool, then place in a round baking dish.

2. Sprinkle the sponge base with the schnapps if using. Wash the raspberries, reserving some for the decoration, then purée the rest. Spread the raspberry purée on the sponge base.

3. Stir together the cream cheese, mascarpone, sugar and vanilla essence to make a smooth mixture. Beat the cream until stiff, then reserve 4 tablespoons for decoration and gently fold the rest into the mixture. Spread this mixture over the raspberry purée. Chill for about 4 hours in the refrigerator.

4. Before serving, decorate with the reserved whipped cream and raspberries.

   TIP
   This raspberry tiramisu can easily be prepared the day before serving.

NUTRITIONAL VALUES PER PORTION:

825 Cal • 23 g protein • 48 g fat • 72 g carbohydrate

Basic recipe Sponge Cake

**MAKES 12 SLICES
   (1 LOOSE-BOTTOMED TIN
   28 CM/11 IN DIAMETER)**

3 eggs
3 tbsp hot water
155 g (5 oz) sugar
a few drops vanilla essence
150 g (5 oz) gluten-free plain flour
butter for greasing

PREPARATION about 20 mins
BAKING about 25 mins

1. Preheat the oven to 200°C (390°F)/175°C (345°F) fan-forced (middle shelf). Line the tin with baking paper and then grease. Beat the eggs with the water until foamy, then add the sugar and the vanilla essence, a little at a time. Sift the flour over the top and quickly fold in.

2. Spread the dough evenly in the tin. Bake in the oven for about 20–25 minutes. Remove from the tin and turn onto the cake rack. Remove the baking paper and leave to cool.

   VARIATIONS
   To make an Almond Sponge, replace the flour with 150 g (5 oz) ground almonds and 50 g (1⅔ oz) cornflour.
   To make a Chocolate Sponge, replace 2 tablespoons flour with 2 tablespoons cocoa.

   TIP
   This sponge base is a real all-rounder – it makes the ideal base for all sorts of fruit fillings and is also excellent for cream cakes or combinations of fruit and cream.

NUTRITIONAL VALUES PER PORTION:

120 Cal • 2 g protein • 2 g fat • 24 g carbohydrate

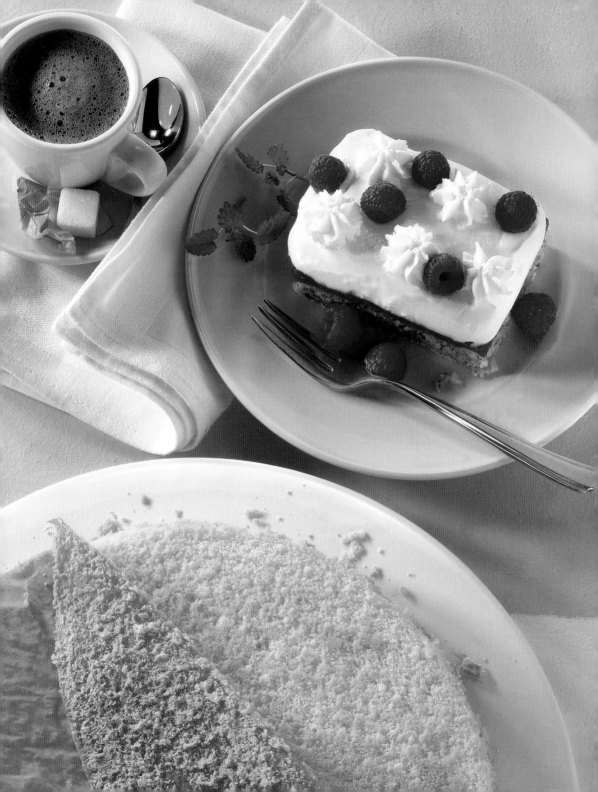

Raspberry Cream Cake

**MAKES 12 SLICES
(1 LOOSE-BOTTOMED TIN
28 CM/11 IN DIAMETER)**

butter for greasing

1 basic recipe Sponge Cake or
　Almond Sponge (see page 72)

1 tsp gelatine powder

750 g (1½ lb) raspberries

100 g (3⅓ oz) sugar

500 g (1 lb) low-fat cream cheese

400 g (13 oz) cream

PREPARATION about 40 mins

CHILLING about 4 hrs

1. Line the tin with baking paper and lightly grease. Bake a sponge cake or almond sponge following the basic recipe.

2. Soak the gelatine according to the packet instructions and leave to swell. In a saucepan, heat, but do not boil the gelatine. Wash the raspberries. Reserve a few for decoration; purée the rest. Stir together with the sugar and the cream cheese. Stir 2–3 tablespoons of the cream cheese mixture into the dissolved gelatine, then stir the gelatine into the cream cheese mixture.

3. Beat the cream until stiff; reserving 4 tablespoons for the decoration. Stir the rest of the cream into the mixture. Place a cake ring around the sponge base. Fill with the mixture. Chill the cake for 4 hours or overnight in the refrigerator until firm.

4. Just before serving, decorate the cake with the reserved raspberries and a few swirls of whipped cream.

TIP

This cake tastes just as delicious if you use frozen instead of fresh raspberries.

NUTRITIONAL VALUES PER PORTION:

360 Cal • 13 g protein • 19 g fat • 34 g carbohydrate

Cheesecake without base

**MAKES 12 SLICES
(1 LOOSE-BOTTOMED TIN
28 CM/11 IN DIAMETER)**

butter for greasing

1 untreated lemon

200 g (6½ oz) soft butter

200 g (6½ oz) sugar

4 eggs

750 g (1½ lb) low-fat cream cheese

1 tbsp polenta

gluten-free instant vanilla custard
　powder (made with 500 ml/
　16 fl oz/2 cups milk as per packet
　instructions)

PREPARATION about 30 mins

BAKING about 1 hr

1. Preheat the oven to 220°C (430°F)/200°C (390°F) fan-forced (middle shelf). Line the tin with baking paper and lightly grease. Wash the lemon under hot water, then pat it dry. Grate the zest, then squeeze out the juice.

2. Beat the butter with the sugar until foamy. Separate the eggs. Add the egg yolks, lemon juice and zest and thoroughly combine with the other ingredients.

3. Stir in the cream cheese, the polenta and the custard. Whisk the egg whites until stiff and fold in. Pour the mixture into the prepared tin.

4. Bake the cake in the oven. After 30 minutes reduce the temperature to 200°C (390°F)/175°C (345°F) fan-forced (middle shelf) and continue baking. After another 20 minutes cover the cake with aluminium foil so it doesn't brown too much. Leave in the tin to cool completely.

VARIATIONS

Add some drained sour cherries (from the jar) to the cream cheese mixture and bake. Sultanas also go very well with the cream cheese mixture.

NUTRITIONAL VALUES PER PORTION:

295 Cal • 11 g protein • 17 g fat • 25 g carbohydrate

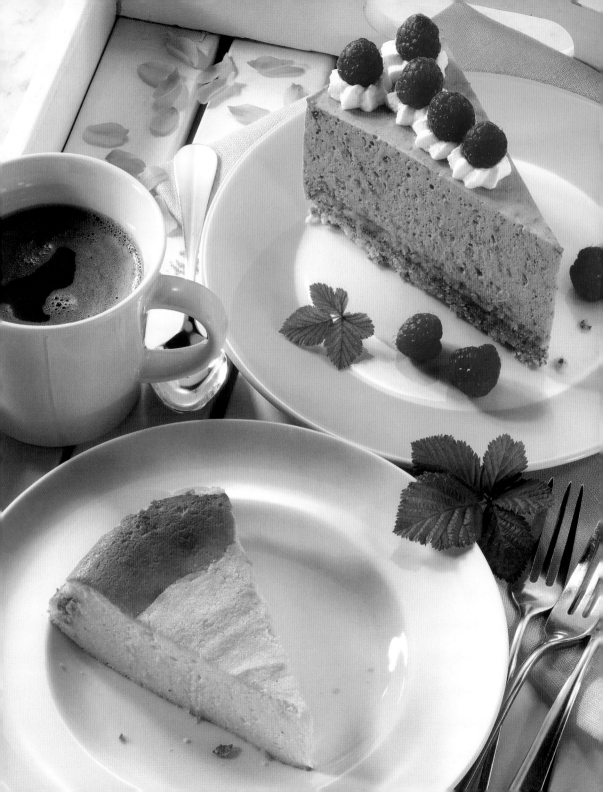

Fruity Walnut Muffins

**MAKES 12 MUFFINS
(1 TRAY WITH 12 HOLES)**

butter for greasing

200 g (6½ oz) cherries (fresh
  or from the jar)

60 g (2 oz) walnut kernels

140 g (4½ oz) gluten-free plain flour

120 g (4 oz) buckwheat flour

3 tsp cream of tartar

½ tsp cinnamon

1 egg

180 g (5¾ oz) raw sugar

100 ml (3 fl oz/½ cup) rapeseed oil

a few drops vanilla essence

250 g (8 oz) yoghurt

PREPARATION about 30 mins

BAKING about 25 mins

1. Preheat the oven to 200°C (390°F)/175°C (345°F) fan-forced (middle shelf). Grease the muffin tray or line the holes with paper cups.

2. Wash and stone the cherries, finely chop the flesh. Place in a sieve to drain. Chop the walnuts. Sift the flour into a bowl and combine well with the buckwheat flour, cream of tartar, cinnamon and the chopped walnuts.

3. Crack the egg into a bowl and whisk lightly. Stir in the sugar, oil, vanilla essence and yoghurt. Quickly stir in the flour mixture. Fold in the chopped cherries.

4. Fill the batter into the holes in the muffin tray. Place the tray in the oven and bake for about 20–25 minutes until golden. Leave to cool for 5 minutes. Remove the muffins from the tray and place them on a cake rack.

VARIATIONS

Instead of using cherries, the muffins can also be made with raspberries, blueberries, strawberries or any other fruit in season.

NUTRITIONAL VALUES PER PORTION:

255 Cal • 3 g protein • 10 g fat • 37 g carbohydrate

Chocolate and Almond Muffins

**MAKES 12 MUFFINS
(1 TRAY WITH 12 HOLES)**

butter for greasing

100 g (3⅓ oz) softened butter

80 g (2¾ oz) raw sugar

1 pinch salt

a few drops vanilla essence

3 eggs

100 g (3⅓ oz) dark chocolate

100 g (3⅓ oz) ground almonds

80 g (2¾ oz) gluten-free plain flour
  (alternatively cornflour)

1 tsp cream of tartar

200 g (6½ oz) chocolate icing

PREPARATION about 30 mins

BAKING about 25 mins

1. Preheat the oven to 200°C (390°F)/175°C (345°F) fan-forced (middle shelf). Grease the muffin tin or place paper cups in the holes.

2. Beat the butter with the sugar, salt and vanilla essence until foamy. Whisk the eggs and stir in, a little at a time. Grate the chocolate or melt it in a bain-marie. Combine with the almonds, flour and cream of tartar, and stir into the batter.

3. Pour the batter into the muffin holes and bake in the oven for about 25 minutes. Leave to cool for 5 minutes.

4. Melt the chocolate icing in a bain-marie. Lift the muffins out of the tin and place them close together on a baking rack. Pour over the melted chocolate icing and leave to cool.

VARIATION

For festive muffins, simply add 1 heaped teaspoon ginger-bread spice to the muffin batter and decorate the baked muffins with little marzipan stars.

NUTRITIONAL VALUES PER PORTION:

315 Cal • 5 g protein • 23 g fat • 25 g carbohydrate

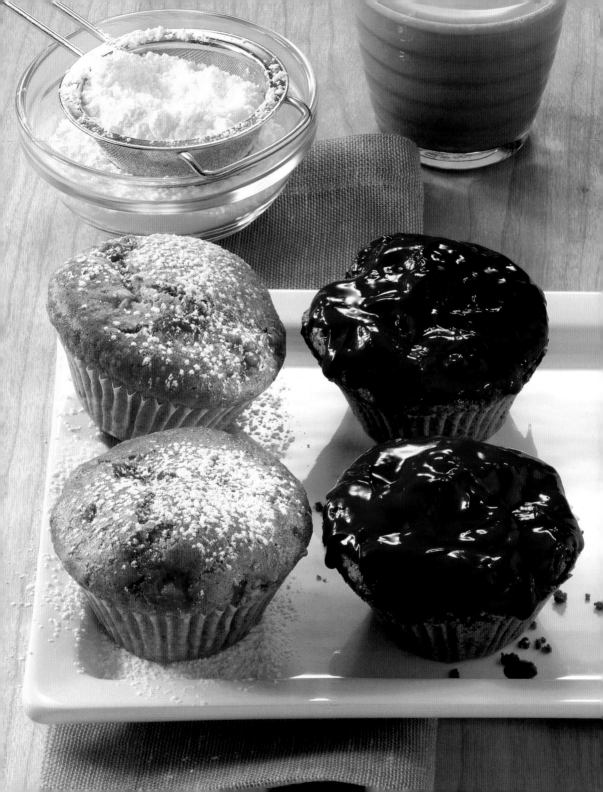

Coconut & Orange Muffins

**MAKES 12 MUFFINS
(1 TRAY WITH 12 HOLES)**
FOR THE BATTER
butter for greasing
100 g (3⅓ oz) raw marzipan
150 g (5 oz) soft butter
80 g (2¾ oz) sugar
4 eggs
1 pinch salt
1 tsp grated zest of 1 untreated lemon
50 g (1⅔ oz) candied orange zest
125 g (4 oz) grated coconut
2 tbsp cornflour (cornstarch)
FOR THE ICING
125 g (4 oz) icing sugar
2-3 tbsp lemon or orange juice
1 tsp grated orange zest

PREPARATION about 30 mins
BAKING about 25 mins

1. Preheat the oven to 200°C (390°F)/175°C (345°F) fan-forced (middle shelf). Grease the muffin tin or line the holes with paper cups.

2. Cut the marzipan into small pieces and beat with the butter and sugar until foamy. Stir in the eggs, salt and lemon zest. Very finely chop the candied orange zest, then fold into the batter together with the grated coconut and the cornflour.

3. Pour the batter into the muffin holes and bake for 20–25 minutes until golden.

4. Lift the muffins out of the tin. Dissolve the icing sugar with the juice and brush the muffins with the mixture while still hot. Sprinkle the grated zest over the muffins. Place the muffins on a baking rack to cool completely.

TIP
You can create particularly decorative zest strips with a so-called zester. This kitchen utensil allows you to peel the orange zest in long, very fine strips. Make sure you use an untreated orange or clean it thoroughly under hot water.

NUTRITIONAL VALUES PER PORTION:
305 Cal • 4 g protein • 21 g fat • 26 g carbohydrate

Almond Slice

MAKES 20 SLICES (1 TRAY)
FOR THE PASTRY BASE
200 ml (7 fl oz/¾ cup) cream
200 g (6 ½ oz) sugar
1 pinch salt
3 eggs
400 g (13 oz) gluten-free plain flour
1 tbsp cream of tartar
FOR THE TOPPING
150 g (5 oz) butter
3 tbsp honey
1 cup sugar
a few drops vanilla essence
200 g (6½ oz) flaked almonds

PREPARATION about 35 mins
BAKING about 30 mins

1. Preheat the oven to 200°C (390°F)/175°C (345°F) fan-forced (middle shelf). Line a tray with baking paper. Beat the cream, sugar and salt until foamy. Stir in the eggs, one at a time. Combine the flour and the cream of tartar and add to the mixture. Mix all the ingredients together. Place the dough in the tray and bake in the oven for 12 minutes.

2. For the topping, heat the butter together with the honey, sugar and vanilla essence. Add the flaked almonds and bring to the boil. Spread this mixture over the prepared pastry base; bake for a further 12–15 minutes.

TIP
You can use the empty plastic container from the cream in this recipe for measuring the flour and the sugar.

NUTRITIONAL VALUES PER PORTION:
315 Cal • 5 g protein • 16 g fat • 40 g carbohydrate

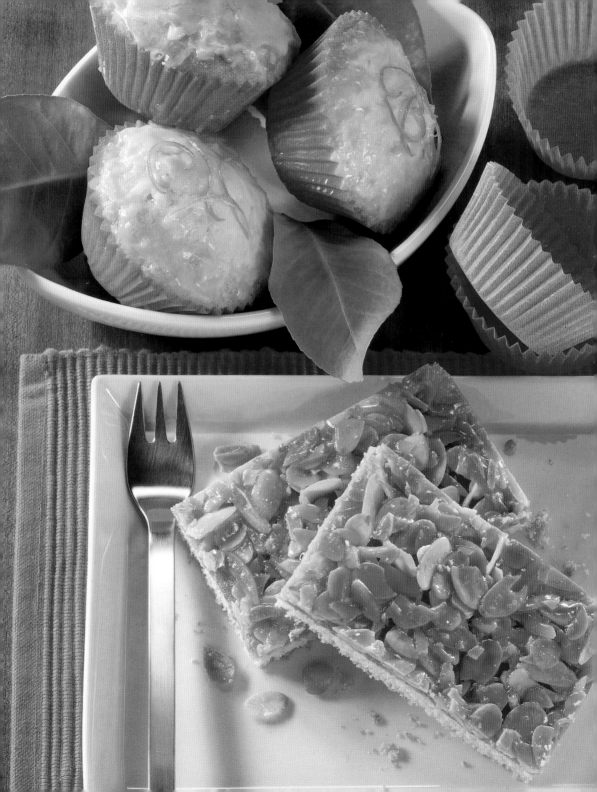

Espresso Cake

MAKES 16 PIECES
(1 LOAF TIN 30 CM/12 IN)

200 g (6½ oz) butter
250 ml (8 fl oz/1 cup) cooled
  espresso
250 g (8 oz) gluten-free plain flour
1½ tbsp cream of tartar
150 g (5 oz) dark chocolate
175 g (5⅔ oz) sugar
1 pinch salt
1 pinch cinnamon
200 g (6½ oz) ground hazelnuts
4 eggs
icing sugar for dusting
PREPARATION about 30 mins
BAKING about 1 hr

1. Preheat the oven to 200°C (390°F)/180°C (355°F) fan-forced (middle shelf). Line the loaf tin with baking paper. Melt the butter in a saucepan and leave to cool. Prepare the espresso and leave to cool.

2. Sift the flour and the cream of tartar into a bowl. Grate the chocolate. Add to the flour together with the sugar, salt, cinnamon and the nuts. Beat the eggs and stir into the batter together with the liquid butter and the espresso.

3. Fill the liquid batter into the loaf tin. Bake the cake in the oven for about 1 hour.

4. Check with a toothpick if the cake is ready. Leave it in the tin for 5 minutes to cool a little, then tip it onto a cake rack and peel away the baking paper. Dust the cake with icing sugar.

TIPS
Alternatively cover the cake with chocolate icing.
Wrap the cake in aluminium foil and keep chilled in the fridge and it will stay nice and moist for several days.

NUTRITIONAL VALUES PER PORTION:
350 Cal • 6 g protein • 25 g fat • 28 g carbohydrate

Buckwheat Cake

MAKES 12 SLICES
(1 LOOSE-BOTTOMED TIN
26 CM/10 IN DIAMETER)

butter for greasing
250 g (8 oz) soft butter
200 g (6½ oz) raw sugar
6 eggs
250 g (8 oz) buckwheat flour
250 g (8 oz) ground almonds
1½ tbsp cream of tartar
400 g (13 oz) frozen raspberries
icing sugar for dusting
PREPARATION about 35 mins
BAKING about 50 mins

1. Preheat the oven to 200°C (390°F)/175°C (345°F) fan-forced (middle shelf). Line the tin with baking paper and lightly grease.

2. Beat the butter with 150 g (5 oz) sugar until foamy. Separate the eggs. Stir in the egg yolks, one at a time. Combine the buckwheat flour with the almonds and the cream of tartar, then stir into the mixture. The dough should be very firm. Thaw the raspberries and leave to drain in a sieve.

3. Beat the egg whites with the remaining cane sugar until stiff, then fold them into the dough. Fill the dough into the tin and bake in the oven for 50 minutes. Using a skewer check if the cake is ready. Remove the cake from the tin and place on a rack to cool.

4. Horizontally cut the cake in half, spread the bottom half with the raspberries and re-assemble the cake. Dust with icing sugar.

VARIATION
For a change, why not replace the ground almonds with ground hazelnuts?

NUTRITIONAL VALUES PER PORTION:
548 Cal • 10 g protein • 33 g fat • 54 g carbohydrate

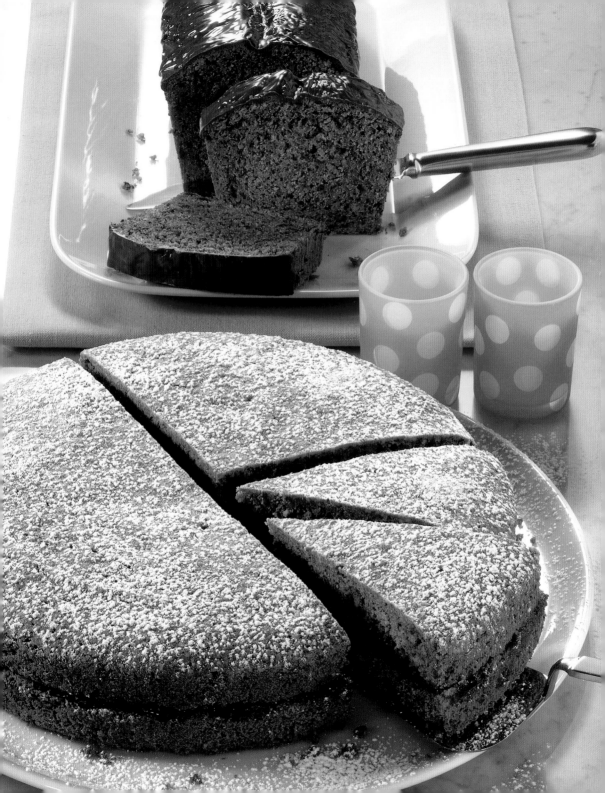

French Cherry Gâteau

MAKES 12 SLICES
(1 LOOSE-BOTTOMED TIN
28 CM/11 IN DIAMETER)

butter for greasing

700 g (1 lb 6 oz) sour cherries
(from the jar)

100 g (3⅓ oz) dark chocolate

200 g (6½ oz) soft butter

150 g (5 oz) raw sugar

4 eggs

125 g (4 oz) gluten-free plain flour

1 tsp cream of tartar

2 tsp rum (if desired)

1 tsp cinnamon

125 g (4 oz) ground hazelnuts

1 pinch salt

icing sugar for dusting

PREPARATION about 40 mins

BAKING about 45 mins

1. Preheat the oven to 220°C (430°F)/200°C (390°F) fan-forced (middle shelf). Line the tin with baking paper, lightly grease. Drain the sour cherries. Grate the chocolate.

2. Beat the butter with the sugar until foamy. Separate the eggs. Stir in the egg yolks, one at a time. Combine the flour with the cream of tartar and stir into the mixture with the rum, cinnamon, nuts and grated chocolate.

3. Beat the egg whites with the salt until stiff, then fold into the dough. Fill the dough into the tin and spread the cherries on top, lightly pressing them into the dough. Bake the gâteau for about 45 minutes.

4. Remove from the tin and place on a rack to cool. Dust with icing sugar before serving.

TIP

You can bake this cake a day ahead of time and it will stay fresh.

NUTRITIONAL VALUES PER PORTION:

390 Cal • 5 g protein • 27 g fat • 33 g carbohydrate

Lemon Cake

MAKES 12 SLICES
(1 LOOSE-BOTTOMED TIN
26 CM/10 IN DIAMETER)

butter for greasing

200 g (6½ oz) soft butter

200 g (6½ oz) sugar

4 eggs

1 tbsp grated zest of 1 untreated lemon

250 g (8 oz) gluten-free plain flour

2 tsp cream of tartar

1 pinch salt

4 lemons

100 g (3⅓ oz) icing sugar

PREPARATION about 30 mins

BAKING about 35 mins

1. Preheat the oven to 200°C (390°F)/180°C (355°F) fan-forced (middle shelf). Line the tin with baking paper and lightly grease. Beat the butter with the sugar until foamy. Separate the eggs, then stir in the egg yolks, one at a time, with the lemon zest. Sift the flour and the cream of tartar over the mixture and stir in.

2. Beat the egg whites with the salt until stiff and gently fold them into the dough. Fill the dough into the tin and smooth the top. Bake in the oven for 30–35 minutes until golden.

3. Squeeze the lemons and dissolve the icing sugar in the juice. Using a kebab stick or a skewer, make many holes in the cake while it is still hot. Brush the lemon syrup over the cake until it has soaked up nearly all the liquid. Place the cake on a rack to cool completely.

TIP

This is a very moist cake and it will still be tasty after a few days - if it doesn't disappear before then.

NUTRITIONAL VALUES PER PORTION:

340 Cal • 3 g protein • 17 g fat • 44 g carbohydrate

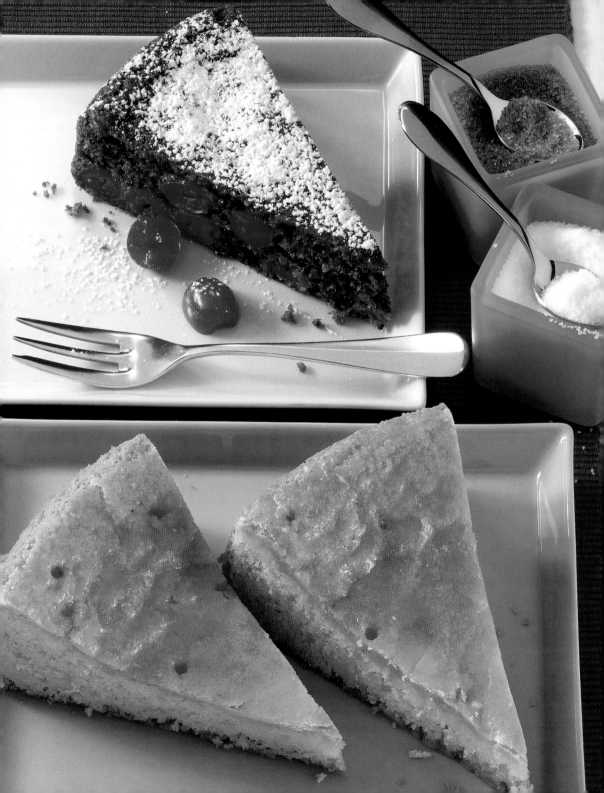

Swiss Carrot Cake

**MAKES 12 SLICES
(1 LOOSE-BOTTOMED TIN
26 CM/10 IN DIAMETER)**

FOR THE DOUGH

butter for greasing

5 eggs

200 g (6½ oz) sugar

1 pinch salt

1 pinch cinnamon

1 pinch ground cloves

4 tsp kirsch or schnapps
(if desired)

200 g (6½ oz) carrots

50 g (1⅔ oz) potato flour or
cornflour (cornstarch)

1 tsp cream of tartar

120 g (4 oz) ground almonds

120 g (4 oz) ground hazelnuts

50 g (1⅔ oz) gluten-free
breadcrumbs

FOR THE ICING

200 g (6½ oz) icing sugar

2 tbsp lemon juice

2 tbsp kirsch or lemon juice

gluten-free marzipan carrots
for decorating

PREPARATION about 40 mins

BAKING about 45 mins

1. Preheat the oven to 200°C (390°F)/175°C (345°F) fan-forced (middle shelf). Line a tin with baking paper and lightly grease. Separate the eggs. Whisk the egg yolks with half the sugar, the salt, cinnamon, cloves and kirsch (if using) until foamy.

2. Clean and peel the carrots, then finely grate them. Combine the starch with the cream of tartar. Add to the carrots with the almonds, nuts and breadcrumbs, then combine well.

3. Whisk the egg whites with the remaining sugar until stiff and fold into the dough. Fill the dough into the tin and smooth. Bake in the oven for about 40–45 minutes. Remove the cake from the tin and place on a rack to cool.

4. Dissolve the icing sugar in the lemon juice and kirsch to make a thick icing. Evenly brush all over the cake once cooled. Decorate with marzipan carrots.

TIPS

This delicious Carrot Cake can be baked one or two days ahead of time – it will stay wonderfully moist.

If you cannot find any ready-made gluten-free marzipan carrots, simply combine raw marzipan with icing sugar and red and yellow food colouring. Shape the mixture into small carrots. To make the green leaves on top of the carrots you can use small pieces of pistachio.

NUTRITIONAL VALUES PER PORTION:
355 Cal • 7 g protein • 16 g fat • 45 g carbohydrate

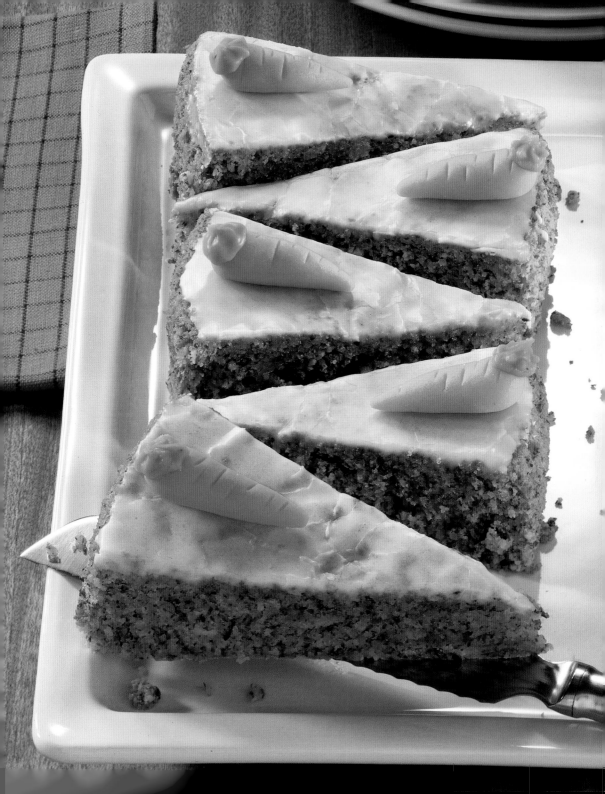

Almond Cake

**MAKES 12 SLICES
(1 LOOSE-BOTTOMED TIN
28 CM/11 IN DIAMETER)**

butter for greasing

6 eggs

1 pinch salt

250 g (8 oz) icing sugar

a few drops vanilla essence

1 pinch cinnamon

1 tbsp grated zest
  of 1 untreated lemon

250 g (8 oz) ground almonds

½ tsp cream of tartar

a few drops lemon juice

melted chocolate for glazing or icing
  sugar for dusting

PREPARATION about 30 mins

BAKING about 50 mins

1. Preheat the oven to 200°C (390°F)/175°C (345°F) fan-forced (middle shelf). Line the tin with baking paper and lightly grease. Separate the eggs. Beat the egg yolks with the salt and the icing sugar until foamy. Add vanilla essence, cinnamon and the grated lemon zest. Combine the almonds with the cream of tartar and carefully fold in. Whisk the egg whites with a few drops of lemon juice until stiff, then carefully fold in.

2. Fill the dough into the tin and bake the cake in the oven for about 50 minutes. Place on a rack to cool. Drizzle with melted chocolate or dust with icing sugar before serving.

VARIATION

This almond cake is also delicious with a chocolate icing. You can easily make this yourself: warm 150 g (5 oz) milk chocolate with 2 tablespoons cream in a bain-marie (or a heatproof bowl set over a saucepan with boiling water). Alternatively, simply use a ready-made icing.

To create another delicious combination, first leave the chocolate icing to dry a little, then sprinkle with dry-roasted flaked almonds.

NUTRITIONAL VALUES PER PORTION:
255 Cal • 7 g protein • 15 g fat • 24 g carbohydrate

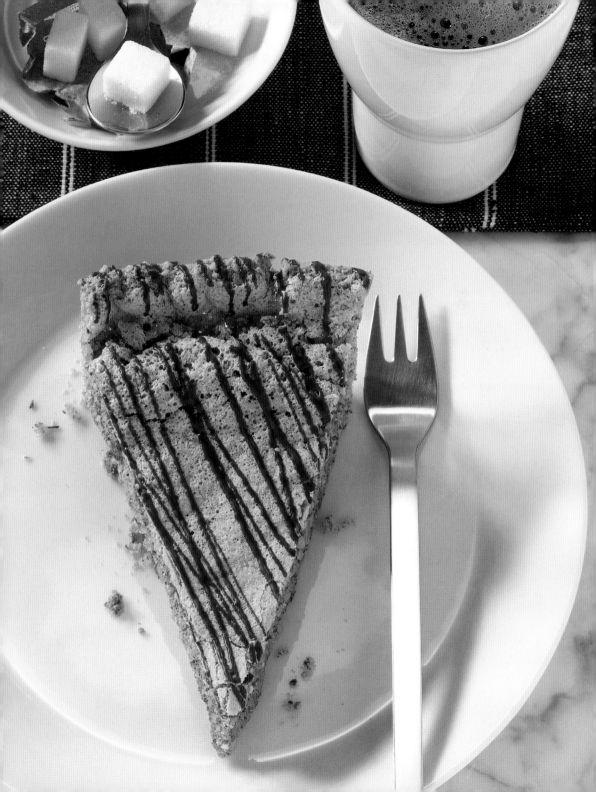

Basic recipe Shortcrust Pastry

**MAKES 12 SLICES
(1 LOOSE-BOTTOMED TIN
28 CM/11 IN DIAMETER)**

butter for greasing

200 g (6½ oz) gluten-free plain flour

60 g (2 oz) sugar

1 pinch salt, 1 egg

90 g (3 oz) cold butter

flour for the work surface

PREPARATION about 20 mins

CHILLING about 1 hr

1. Line the tin with baking paper and lightly grease.

2. Sift the flour onto a board. Add sugar, salt and the egg. Put on small pats of the cold butter. Quickly knead all the ingredients into a dough that can be rolled out. Add more flour if needed. Wrap in cling film and chill for about 1 hour in the refrigerator.

3. Dust the work surface with flour. Cut the dough into slices and place these close to each other on the work surface, then roll out as a sheet. Place the dough into the tin, forming a 2–3 cm (¾–1¼ in) rim.

4. Cover with a topping of your choice (see below and page 90) and bake as per the recipe instructions.

> **VARIATIONS**
>
> This pastry base is also ideal for making delicious apple, rhubarb, redcurrant, gooseberry and cheesecake.

> **TIPS**
>
> You can roll out the dough straight onto the baking paper and then chill it after placing it in the tin. In that case it is sufficient to chill the short pastry base for 30 minutes instead of 1 hour.
> Add 1 teaspoon fibre husk (psyllium) to the flour. It will make the pastry dough smooth and also easier to work.

NUTRITIONAL VALUES PER PORTION:

140 Cal • 1 g protein • 7 g fat • 19 g carbohydrate

Rhubarb Cake with custard topping

**MAKES 12 SLICES
(1 LOOSE-BOTTOMED TIN
28 CM/11 IN DIAMETER)**

1 basic recipe Shortcrust
    Pastry (above)

FOR THE TOPPING

butter for greasing

gluten-free instant vanilla custard powder
    (made with 500 ml/16 fl oz/2 cups
    milk as per packet instructions)

500 ml (16 fl oz/2 cups) milk

600 g (1 lb 3 oz) rhubarb

125 g (4 oz) butter

3 tbsp sugar, 3 eggs

PREPARATION about 40 mins

BAKING about 45 mins

1. Prepare the short pastry according to the basic recipe. After chilling, preheat the oven to 200°C (390°F)/180°C (355°F) fan-forced (middle shelf). Line the tin with baking paper, lightly grease.

2. Cook the custard with the milk and leave to cool. Wash, thinly peel and dice the rhubarb, about 2 cm (¾ in) dice, then blanch in boiling water. Drain.

3. Roll out the pastry and place it in the tin, forming an edge of 2–3 cm (¾–1¼ in). Place the drained pieces of rhubarb on top of the dough. Bake the cake in the oven for 20 minutes.

4. Meanwhile, beat the butter with the sugar until foamy. Separate the eggs. Stir the egg yolks into about two-thirds of the vanilla custard once it has cooled a little. (The butter and the custard should have roughly the same temperature.) Beat the egg whites until stiff, then fold in. Spread the mixture on top of the cake and bake for another 20–25 minutes until golden. Leave in the tin for 10 minutes to cool a little, then place on a wire rack to cool completely. Serve fresh.

NUTRITIONAL VALUES PER PORTION:

300 Cal • 4 g protein • 19 g fat • 28 g carbohydrate

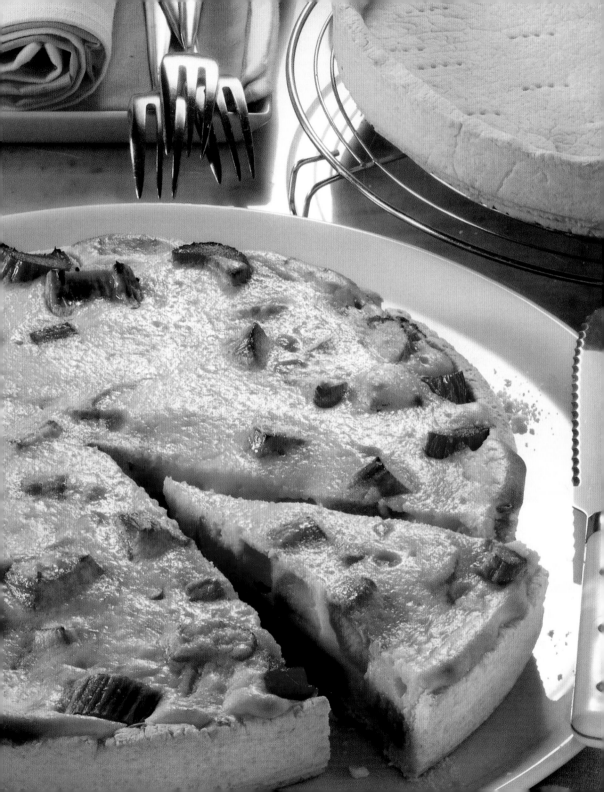

Gooseberry Cake

MAKES 12 SLICES
(1 LOOSE-BOTTOMED TIN
28 CM/11 IN DIAMETER)

butter for greasing

1 basic recipe Shortcrust Pastry
  (see page 88)

5 egg whites

200 g (6½ oz) sugar

125 g (4 oz) ground almonds

500 g (1 lb) gooseberries

PREPARATION about 20 mins

CHILLING about 1 hr

BAKING about 50 mins

1. Prepare the pastry base according to the basic recipe. Preheat the oven to 250°C (480°F)/200°C (390°F) fan-forced (middle shelf). Line the tin with baking paper and lightly grease. Roll out the dough, place in the tin. Form a dough edge of about 3 cm (1¼ in).

2. Whisk the egg whites until stiff, then sprinkle in the sugar, a little at a time, while continuing to whisk, until you have a thick mixture. Fold in the almonds.

3. Spread one-third of the mixture onto the dough base. Stir the berries into the remaining mixture, spread on top of the dough and smooth. Bake in the oven for 45–50 minutes, until the cake is just beginning to brown. Leave to cool in the tin for 10 minutes, then on a rack.

TIP

You can also use frozen berries for this recipe. They will not need to be thawed before use.

VARIATION

Instead of the gooseberries, try blueberries in this cake for a different flavour.

NUTRITIONAL VALUES PER PORTION:

295 Cal • 5 g protein • 13 g fat • 41 g carbohydrate

Apple Cake with cinnamon frosting

MAKES 12 SLICES
(1 LOOSE-BOTTOMED TIN
28 CM/11 IN DIAMETER)

butter for greasing

1 basic recipe Short Pastry
  (see page 88)

2 tbsp gluten-free breadcrumbs
  (or ground hazelnuts)

5-6 apples (e.g. Granny Smith or
  Golden Delicious)

2 eggs

100 g (3⅓ oz) sugar

125 g (4 oz) sour cream

1 heaped tsp cinnamon

50 g (1⅔ oz) chopped almonds

PREPARATION about 20 mins

RESTING about 1 hr

BAKING about 50 mins

1. Prepare the Short Pastry base according to the basic recipe. Preheat the oven to 200°C (390°F)/175°C (345°F) fan-forced (middle shelf). Line the tin with baking paper and lightly grease. Roll out the pastry, place it in the tin and sprinkle with the breadcrumbs.

2. Peel and core the apples, then cut into wedges. Place in a fan shape on top of the pastry base. Beat the eggs with the sugar until foamy. Stir in the sour cream and the cinnamon. Add the almonds. Spread the mixture evenly over the apples.

3. Bake in the oven for about 50 minutes. Turn off the oven, leaving the cake inside the oven for another 10 minutes. Leave the cake in the tin to cool for 10 minutes, then remove. Place on a rack to cool completely.

NUTRITIONAL VALUES PER PORTION:

260 Cal • 3 g protein • 12 g fat • 35 g carbohydrate

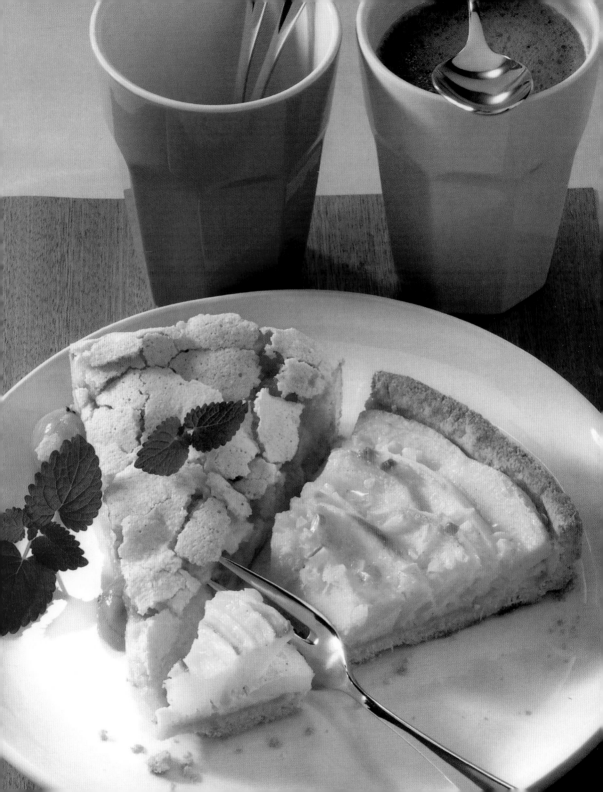

Linzer Torte

**MAKES 12 SLICES
(1 LOOSE-BOTTOMED TIN
28 CM/11 IN DIAMETER)**

butter for greasing

200 g (6½ oz) gluten-free
plain flour

150 g (5 oz) sugar

a few drops vanilla essence

200 g (6½ oz) ground almonds

1 tsp ground cinnamon

1 pinch ground cloves

1 egg

4 tsp kirsch (if desired)

200 g (6½ oz) cold butter

flour for the work surface

200 g (6½ oz) raspberry jam

1 egg yolk

PREPARATION about 40 mins
RESTING about 1 hr
BAKING about 1 hr

1. Grease the baking tin. Combine the flour, sugar, vanilla essence, almonds, cinnamon and cloves on a board and make a well in the middle. Crack the egg into it and add the kirsch (if using), place the butter around the edge in small pats. Quickly knead everything together with cold hands until you have a smooth dough. Wrap the dough in cling film and chill for about 1 hour in the refrigerator.

2. Preheat the oven to 200°C (390°F)/175°C (345°F) fan-forced (middle shelf). Dust the work surface with flour and roll out half the dough about 5 mm (¼ in) thick. Place the dough in the tin and form a rim of about 1 cm (½ in). Spread with the jam. Roll out the remaining dough and cut out hearts, stars or fancy rounds with a pastry cutter. Place the shapes on top of the cake and brush with the egg yolk.

3. Bake the torte in the oven for about 1 hour. Remove from the tin and leave to cool completely on a rack.

TIPS

Wrap the Linzer Torte in aluminium foil and it will easily keep for 1–2 weeks.
In the pre-Christmas period, cut out stars instead of hearts or rounds to add a festive touch.

VARIATION

Instead of the raspberry jam, use some apricot jam to make your next Linzer Torte for a tasty variation.

NUTRITIONAL VALUES PER PORTION:
300 Cal • 1 g protein • 15 g fat • 37 g carbohydrate

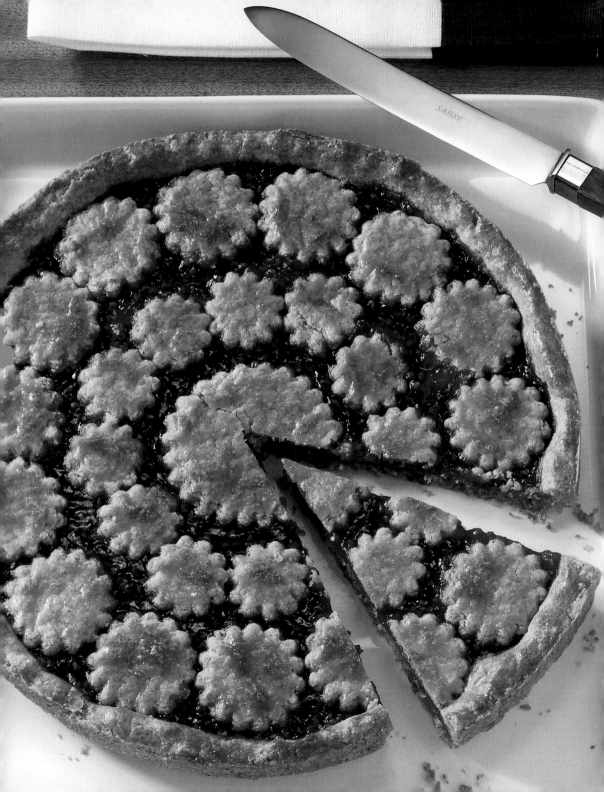

Butter Biscuits

MAKES ABOUT 50 BISCUITS

150 g (5 oz) soft butter

150 g (5 oz) icing sugar

a few drops vanilla essence

1 egg

70 g (2½ oz) ground almonds

250 g (8 oz) gluten-free plain flour

flour for the work surface

PREPARATION about 30 mins

CHILLING about 1 hr

BAKING about 8 mins

1. Line the baking tray with baking paper. Beat butter, icing sugar and vanilla essence until pale in colour. Add the egg and continue beating for 2 minutes. Knead in the almonds and the flour, a little at a time. At this point the dough will be a little softer than it needs to be for rolling out, but it will become firmer. Wrap the dough in cling film and chill for about 1 hour in the refrigerator.

2. Preheat the oven to 220°C (430°F)/200°C (390°F) fan-forced (middle shelf). Dust the work surface with flour and roll out the dough about 3mm (⅛ in) thick. Use pastry cutters to cut out various shapes and place them on the trays. Bake in the oven for about 8 minutes until golden. Remove the biscuits from the tray with the paper and leave to cool.

TIP

To make the dough much easier to work with, knead 1 teaspoon fibre husk (psyllium) into the dough.

VARIATIONS

Decorate the biscuits with icing and gluten-free multi-coloured sprinkles (100s and 1000s).

JAM BISCUITS

Cut out same-sized, small round biscuits from the dough. For half the biscuits, cut out smaller round holes in their middle. After baking, brush the whole biscuits with redcurrant jam, then place the biscuits with holes on top. Dust the jam biscuits with icing sugar.

MACAROONS

Place a small dab of almond paste in the middle of the biscuits and bake. This will taste delicious and also look pretty.

LINZER COOKIES

Shape the dough into small balls (about 2 cm/¾ in). Using the stem of a wooden cooking spoon press a small hollow in the middle of each biscuit, then fill this with raspberry jam.

BISCUIT CREAMS

Cut out round biscuits in 3 different sizes and stack them after baking with nougat cream. Dust with icing sugar.

NUTRITIONAL VALUES PER PORTION:

60 Cal • 1 g protein • 3 g fat • 7 g carbohydrate

Fancy Pistachio Fingers

MAKES ABOUT 50 FINGERS

flour for the work surface

200 g (6½ oz) gluten-free plain flour

170 g (5½ oz) cold butter

125 g (4 oz) sugar

a few drops vanilla essence

100 g (3⅓ oz) ground pistachios

100 g (3⅓ oz) ground almonds

3 drops bitter almond oil

200 g (6½ oz) chocolate icing
(ready-made)

20 g (⅔ oz) chopped pistachios

PREPARATION about 40 mins

RISING about 1 hr

BAKING about 10 mins

1. Line the baking trays with baking paper. Sift the flour onto the work surface. Cut the butter into small pieces and add them to flour together with the sugar, vanilla essence, ground pistachios, ground almonds and the bitter almond oil. Quickly knead to make a dough. Add more flour if needed. Wrap in cling film and chill for 1 hour in the refrigerator.

2. Preheat the oven to 190°C (375°F)/170°C (340°F) fan-forced (middle shelf). Dust the work surface with four and roll out the dough to ½ cm (¼ in) thick. Using a pastry cutter or a knife, cut it into fingers of about 6x2 cm (2⅓ by ¾ in). Carefully transfer the fingers to the tray and bake in the oven for 9–10 minutes.

3. Leave the fingers on the tray to cool, otherwise they will break. Brush about half with chocolate icing and sprinkle with the chopped pistachios.

TIP

Store the pistachio fingers in a tin as it will keep them nice and crumbly. These are ideal for tea with guests.

NUTRITIONAL VALUES PER PORTION:

95 Cal • 1 g protein • 6 g fat • 9 g carbohydrate

Lemon Hearts

MAKES ABOUT 40 HEARTS

3 egg yolks

120 g (4 oz) sugar

a few drops vanilla sugar

5 drops lemon flavouring

200 g (6½ oz) ground almonds

icing sugar for the work surface

100 g (3⅓ oz) icing sugar

2-3 tbsp lemon juice

PREPARATION about 30 mins

BAKING about 15 mins

1. Preheat the oven to 180°C (355°F)/160°C (320°F) fan-forced (middle shelf). Line the baking trays with baking paper. Whisk the egg yolks with the sugar, vanilla essence and lemon flavouring until foamy. Add the almonds and knead all the ingredients together until you have a smooth dough.

2. Sprinkle the work surface with icing sugar and roll out the dough about 3 mm thick. Cut out heart shapes and place them on the trays. Bake in the oven for 12–15 minutes.

3. Dissolve the icing sugar in the lemon juice and brush the hearts while still hot with the glaze. Remove the hearts from the trays using the paper and leave to cool.

TIP

You can save eggs if you bake these Lemon Hearts on the same day as other biscuits where egg whites are needed, for example the macaroons on page 98.

NUTRITIONAL VALUES PER PORTION:

55 Cal • 1 g protein • 3 g fat • 6 g carbohydrate

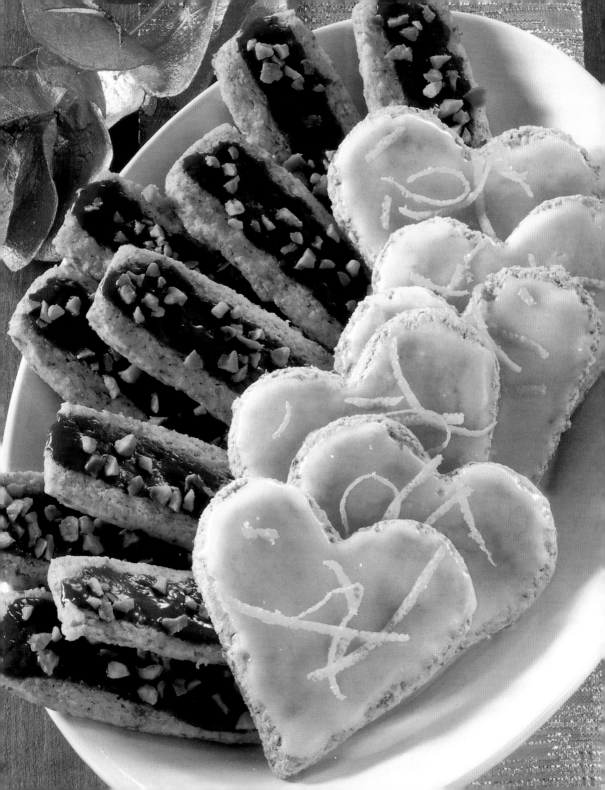

Coconut & Marzipan Macaroons

MAKES ABOUT 50
MACAROONS

150 g (5 oz) desiccated coconut

4 egg whites

300 g (10 oz) marzipan

200 g (6½ oz) icing sugar

1 tsp grated zest
of 1 untreated lemon

1 tbsp rum (or 10 drops
rum flavouring)

5 tbsp sugar

200 g (6½ oz) chocolate icing
(ready-made)

PREPARATION about 40 mins

BAKING about 20 mins

1. Preheat the oven to 100°C (210°F)/80°C (175°F) fan-forced (middle shelf). Line the trays with baking paper. Sprinkle the coconut onto one tray and dry out in the oven for about 15 minutes, then leave to cool. Increase the oven temperature to 180°C (355°F)/160°C (320°F) fan-forced (middle shelf).

2. Whisk the egg whites until stiff. Cut the marzipan into very small pieces and stir into the egg whites together with the icing sugar, lemon zest and rum if using. Add the coconut and stir all the ingredients together to form a viscous mixture.

3. Using two teaspoons, place little heaps of the mixture onto the trays. Sprinkle the macaroons with sugar. Bake them in the oven for about 20 minutes until the tops are golden. Leave to cool completely on a rack.

4. Melt the chocolate icing in a bain-marie and use to decorate the macaroons. Cover about half of each macaroon with the melted chocolate or alternatively pour the couverture into a small freezer bag, cut off a tiny corner and pipe spirals or other patterns onto the macaroons.

NUTRITIONAL VALUES PER PORTION:
90 Cal • 1 g protein • 5 g fat • 11 g carbohydrate

Hazelnut Macaroons

MAKES ABOUT 40
MACAROONS

3 egg whites

1 pinch salt

150 g (5 oz) sugar

250 g (8 oz) ground hazelnuts

PREPARATION about 25 mins

DRYING about 4 hrs

BAKING about 20 mins

1. Line the trays with baking paper. Beat the egg whites with the salt until stiff. Add half the sugar and continue beating until the mixture becomes glossy. Stir in the remaining sugar.

2. Fold the hazelnuts into the egg white mixture. Using two teaspoons, place little heaps of the mixture onto the trays. Leave the macaroons to dry for about 3–4 hours at room temperature.

3. Preheat the oven to 175°C (345°F)/150°C (300°F) fan-forced (middle shelf). Bake the macaroons for about 15–20 minutes. Place on a rack to cool completely.

VARIATIONS

Substitute ground walnuts, almonds or shredded coconut for the ground hazelnuts.

To make different-flavoured macaroons, simply add some ground cinnamon, a few drops of vanilla essence, some bitter almond oil, butter and vanilla flavouring, grated lemon zest or small chocolate pieces for that extra special touch.

NUTRITIONAL VALUES PER PORTION:
57 Cal • 1 g protein • 4 g fat • 4 g carbohydrate

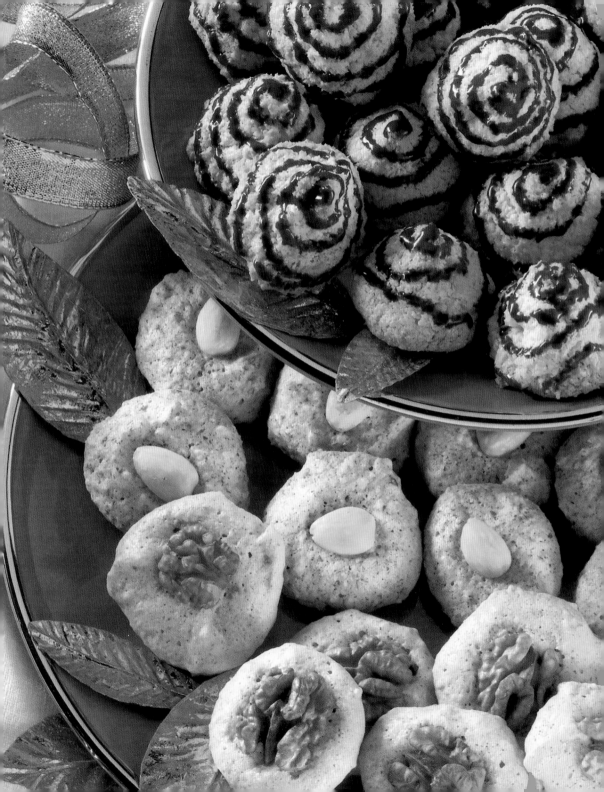

Almond Crescents

MAKES ABOUT 40 CRESCENTS

500 g (1 lb) marzipan

150 g (5 oz) sugar

2 egg whites

1 tbsp grated zest
    of 1 untreated lemon

10 drops bitter almond oil

100 g (3⅓ oz) flaked almonds

200 g (6½ oz) chocolate icing
    (ready-made)

PREPARATION about 30 mins

BAKING about 15 mins

1. Preheat the oven to 200°C (390°F)/175°C (345°F) fan-forced (middle shelf). Line the trays with baking paper. Knead the marzipan with the sugar, egg whites, lemon zest and bitter almond oil to form a dough. Moisten your hands and shape the dough into rolls, about 6 cm (2⅓ in) long. Place the almonds on a plate. Turn the rolls in the almonds, then shape them into crescents.

2. Place the crescents on the trays; bake for 12–15 minutes until golden. Place on a rack to cool completely.

3. Melt the chocolate icing in a bain-marie and dip the ends of the crescents in the melted couverture.

TIPS

You can make the croissants twice the size, if you prefer. If they are this size they will need to bake for about 20 minutes. The crescents will keep for at least 1 week if they are stored in a tin.

VARIATION

Replace the almonds with chopped pistachios.

NUTRITIONAL VALUES PER PORTION:

115 Cal • 2 g protein • 6 g fat • 13 g carbohydrate

Chocolate Slices

MAKES ABOUT 40 SLICES

250 g (8 oz) dark chocolate

250 g (8 oz) soft butter

150 g (5 oz) sugar

6 eggs

250 g (8 oz) ground almonds

3 tbsp gluten-free plain flour
    (or cornflour)

200 g (6½ oz) chocolate icing
    (ready-made)

PREPARATION about 25 mins

BAKING about 45 mins

1. Preheat the oven to 175°C (345°F)/150°C (300°F) fan-forced (middle shelf). Line the tray with baking paper. Melt the chocolate in a bain-marie. Leave to cool a little.

2. Beat the butter with the sugar until pale, then stir in the eggs, one at a time. Stir in the almonds, melted chocolate and flour. Spread the mixture 1½–2 cm (⅔–¾ in) thick onto the prepared tray and bake in the oven for 40–45 minutes. Leave on the tray to cool.

3. Melt the chocolate icing in a bain-marie, then spread over the chocolate slice. Leave the icing to set a little. Cut the chocolate slice into rectangles 4cm x 6 cm (1½ in x 2⅓ in).

TIP

You can replace the ground almonds with ground hazelnuts if you prefer.

NUTRITIONAL VALUES PER PORTION:

170 Cal • 3 g protein • 14 g fat • 9 g carbohydrate

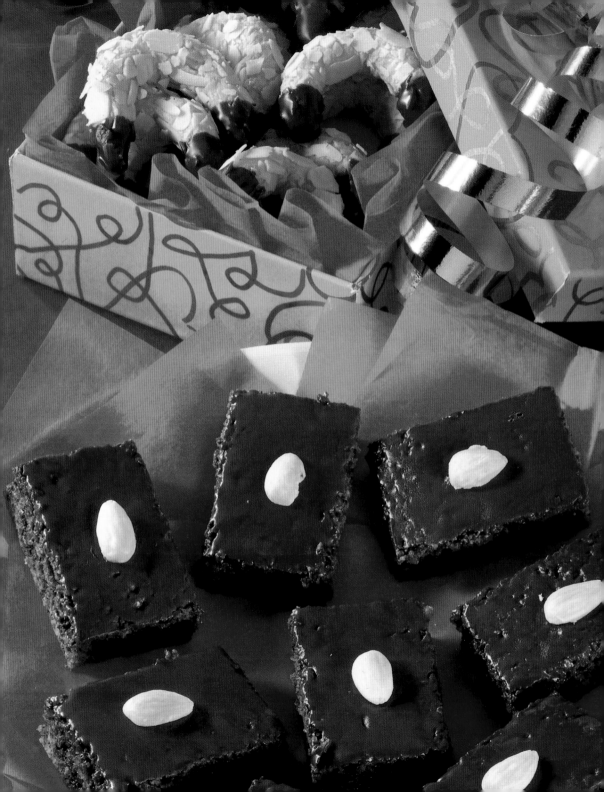

Mini Meringues

MAKES ABOUT 100
MERINGUES

250 g (8 oz) flaked almonds

200 g (6½ oz) sugar

4 egg whites

1 pinch salt

1 tbsp grated orange zest

150 g (5 oz) grated chocolate

PREPARATION about 45 mins

DRYING about 1 hr

BAKING about 20 mins

NUTRITIONAL VALUES PER PORTION:

30 Cal • 1 g protein • 2 g fat • 3 g carbohydrate

1. Line the baking trays with baking paper. In a non-stick frying pan lightly roast the almonds with half the sugar and 2 tablespoons water over a low temperature, stirring constantly. Leave to cool.

2. Whisk the egg whites until stiff, then stir in the remaining sugar, salt and orange zest. Fold in the grated chocolate and almond mixture once cooled. Using a teaspoon, place small heaps of the mixture onto the baking trays. Leave the mini meringues to dry for about 1 hour.

3. Preheat the oven to 175°C (345°F)/160°C (320°F) fan-forced (middle shelf). Bake the mini meringues for about 20 minutes. Remove them from the trays using the paper and leave to cool.

Walnut cookies

MAKES ABOUT 50 COOKIES

100 g (3⅓ oz) dark chocolate

200 g (6½ oz) ground walnuts

50 g (1⅔ oz) ground almonds +
   some for working

200 g (6½ oz) icing sugar

½ tsp cinnamon

½ tsp ground cloves

2 egg whites

1 tbsp kirsch (if liked)

2 tbsp whole cane sugar

50 walnut halves for decorating

PREPARATION about 30 mins

CHILLING about 2 hrs

BAKING about 10 mins

NUTRITIONAL VALUES PER PORTION:

80 Cal • 2 g protein • 6 g fat • 6 g carbohydrate

1. Line the trays with baking paper. Finely grate the chocolate and combine with the walnuts, almonds, icing sugar, cinnamon and cloves.

2. Whisk the egg whites until creamy but not stiff, then stir in the chocolate mixture and the kirsch if using, until you have a firm dough that can be shaped. Add some more almonds to the dough if needed.

3. Sprinkle the work surface with the sugar and shape the dough into 3 rolls of 3 cm (1¼ in) diameter. Wrap separately in cling film and chill for 2 hours in the refrigerator.

4. Preheat the oven to 220°C (430°F)/200°C (390°F) fan-forced (middle shelf). Cut rounds about 1 cm (½ in) thick from the rolls, place them on the trays and decorate each one with a walnut half. Bake in the oven for 8–10 minutes. Remove from the tray using the baking paper and leave to cool.

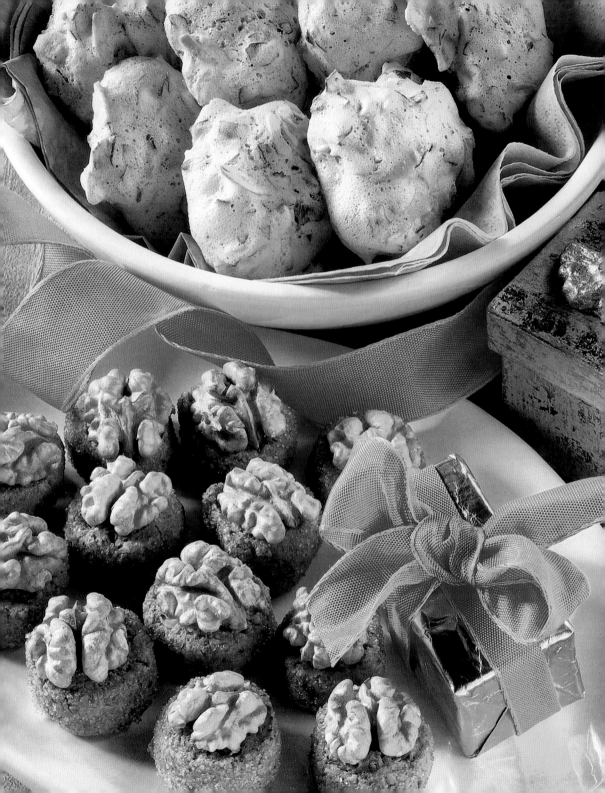

Weekend Bread Rolls

MAKES 12 ROLLS

1 tbsp psyllium (fibre husk)

400 ml (14 fl oz/1¾ cups)
   lukewarm water

500 g (1 lb) gluten-free plain flour

1½ tsp dried yeast

1 tsp sugar

1½ tsp salt

30 g (1 oz) soft butter

1 tbsp apple cider vinegar

poppy seeds, sesame seeds,
   sunflower seeds for sprinkling

PREPARATION about 30 mins

RESTING about 40 mins

BAKING about 30 mins

1. Stir the psyllium into the lukewarm water and leave to swell for 10 minutes. Line the baking tray with baking paper.

2. Combine the flour with the yeast, sugar and salt. Add the fibre husk and water mixture, the butter and the vinegar and knead until you have a smooth dough that easily comes off the edge of the bowl. Add some more flour if needed.

3. Moisten a spatula and use this to divide the dough into 12 even-sized pieces. Moisten your hands, then shape into bread rolls. Place the rolls on the tray and sprinkle with the grains. Gently press the grains into the dough. Leave the dough to rise in the warm oven for about 25–30 minutes (see tips).

4. Remove the tray from the oven. Preheat the oven to 225°C (435°F)/200°C (390°F) fan-forced (middle shelf) for about 30 minutes until golden. After baking leave to cool completely on a rack.

TIPS

Gluten-free dough requires plenty of moisture in order to rise well. The following method has proved successful. Briefly preheat the oven to 50°C (120°F) , then turn it off (about 35°C/95°F). Place the bread rolls on a tray or the bread loaf in the tin into the oven, then place a grate covered with a damp kitchen cloth on top. Before baking, make sure you remove the kitchen cloth! Get a bowl of water ready next to you before you start baking. You can use it to moisten first the spatula and then your hands repeatedly as you shape the rolls.

PSYLLIUM (FIBRE HUSK)

Adding the psyllium makes the dough extra-smooth and improves its rising properties. This makes the dough absorb lots of liquid. It also preserves this moisture better in the gluten-free baked goods so they do not dry out so quickly. Psyllium is a relatively recent arrival in the gluten-free kitchen.

NUTRITIONAL VALUES PER PORTION:
205 Cal • 2 g protein • 6 g fat • 36 g carbohydrate

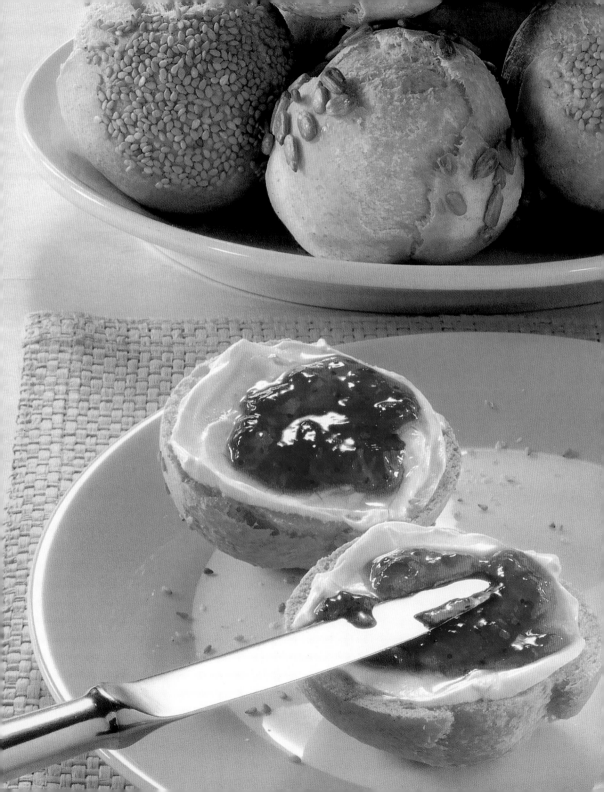

Wholemeal Bread Rolls or wholemeal bread

**MAKES 12 ROLLS OR 1 LOAF
(28 CM/11 IN LONG)**

butter for greasing

500 g (1 lb) gluten-free four-grain bread mix

50 g (1²/₃ oz) linseed (flaxseed)

50 g (1²/₃ oz) rice bran

150 g (5 oz) dried sourdough

1½ tsp dried yeast, 1 tsp sea salt

1 tsp raw sugar

1 tbsp olive oil

550 ml (18 fl oz/2¹/₃ cups) lukewarm water

sunflower seeds to sprinkle

PREPARATION about 30 mins

RISING about 30 mins

BAKING about 30 mins

NUTRITIONAL VALUES PER PORTION:

245 Cal • 7 g protein • 6 g fat • 40 g carbohydrate

1. Line the tray with baking paper or grease the tin. Combine the bread mix with the linseed, rice bran, sourdough, dried yeast, salt and sugar. Add the oil and the water and stir until you have a fairly firm dough.

2. Moisten your hands and shape 12 round rolls and set them on the tray; alternatively, place the dough into a loaf tin. Sprinkle with sunflower seeds and lightly press these into the dough. Leave the rolls or the loaf to rise in the warm oven for about 30 minutes (see Tips on page 104).

3. Remove from the oven. Preheat the oven to 250°C (480°F)/220°C (430°F) fan-forced (middle shelf) and bake for about 10 minutes. Reduce the temperature to 225°C (430°F)/200°C (390°F) fan-forced and bake for another 15–20 minutes. After baking, remove the bread from the tin. Leave the rolls to cool completely on a wire rack.

VARIATION

Sprinkle the dough with sesame seeds, poppy seeds or buckwheat flakes instead of the sunflower seeds.

Yeast-free Bread Rolls

MAKES 10 BREAD ROLLS

250 g (8 oz) gluten-free plain flour

2 tsp cream of tartar

½ tsp salt

150 g (5 oz) low-fat cream cheese

6 tbsp milk

1 small egg

6 tbsp rapeseed oil

poppy seeds, sesame seeds or sunflower seeds for sprinkling

PREPARATION about 20 mins

CHILLING about 30 mins

BAKING about 25 mins

1. Combine the flour with the cream of tartar and the salt. Stir together the cream cheese, milk, egg and oil. Add this to the flour and knead until you have a smooth dough. Add more flour if needed. Wrap the dough in cling film and leave to chill in the refrigerator for 30 minutes.

2. Preheat the oven to 200°C (390°F)/180°C (355°F) fan-forced (middle shelf). Line the baking tray with baking paper. Cut the dough into 10 even parts. Moisten your hands and shape rolls. Sprinkle with poppy, sesame or sunflower seeds and lightly press the seeds into the dough. Make a crossways cut in the top with a sharp knife and place on the tray.

3. Bake the rolls in the oven for about 25 minutes. After baking, leave to cool on a rack.

VARIATION

To make sweet rolls add a pinch salt, 6 tablespoons sugar and 1 teaspoon grated lemon zest to the dough, or add 50 g (1²/₃ oz) raisins. Brush the sweet rolls with egg yolk before baking.

NUTRITIONAL VALUES PER PORTION:

200 Cal • 5 g protein • 10 g fat • 23 g carbohydrate

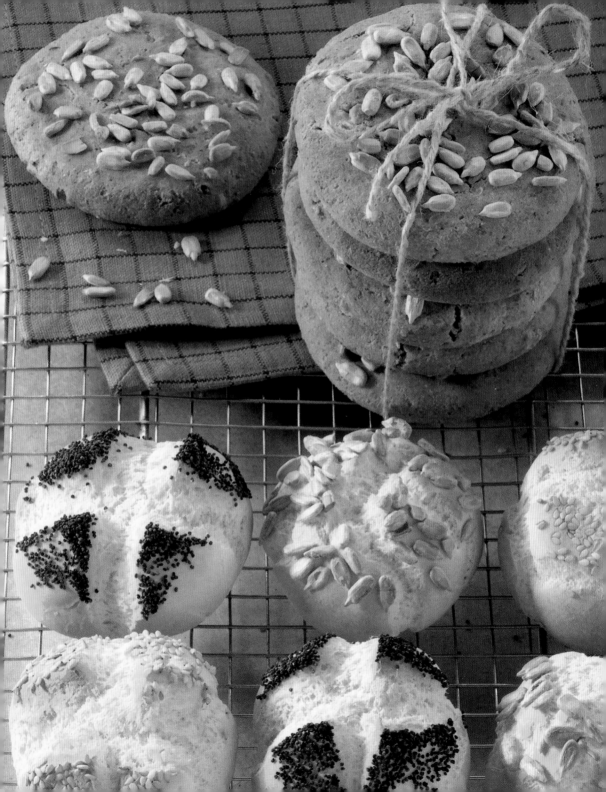

White Bread Rolls or white bread

**MAKES 12 ROLLS OR 1 LOAF
(24 CM/9½ IN LONG)**

butter for greasing

1 tsp psyllium (fibre husk)

450 ml (15 fl oz/1¾ cups) lukewarm
    water

500 g (1 lb) gluten-free bread
    mix for white bread

1½ tsp dried yeast

1 tsp sugar

3 tbsp olive oil

PREPARATION about 20 mins

RISING about 40 mins

BAKING about 50 mins

1. Stir the psyllium into the lukewarm water and leave to swell for 10 minutes. Line the baking tray with baking paper or grease the loaf tin.

2. Combine the flour with the yeast and the sugar. Add 1 tablespoon oil and the psyllium and water, then knead until you have a smooth dough (not too firm) and easy to shape by hand.

3. Moisten your hands and shape 12 even-sized rolls. Place on the tray or place the dough into a loaf tin. Leave the rolls or the bread to rise in a warm oven (see Tips on page 104) for about 30–40 minutes, or until they have doubled in volume.

4. Remove the tray from the oven; then preheat the oven to 225°C (430°F)/200°C (390°F) fan-forced (middle shelf). Bake the rolls or the bread for about 40 minutes. Brush the bread with 2 tablespoons oil and bake for another 10 minutes to finish. After baking, leave to cool on a rack.

TIP

This is an ideal dough for a light and fluffy white bread. You can also use it to bake baguettes (French sticks).

VARIATION

To make sunflower seed rolls, stir 30 g (1 oz) sunflower seeds into the dough. Brush the rolls with a little cream and sprinkle this with more sunflower seeds. Using the palm of your hand, lightly press the seeds into the dough. Bake these delicious sunflower seed rolls for about 30 minutes.

NUTRITIONAL VALUES PER PORTION:
175 Cal • 1 g protein • 3 g fat • 35 g carbohydrate

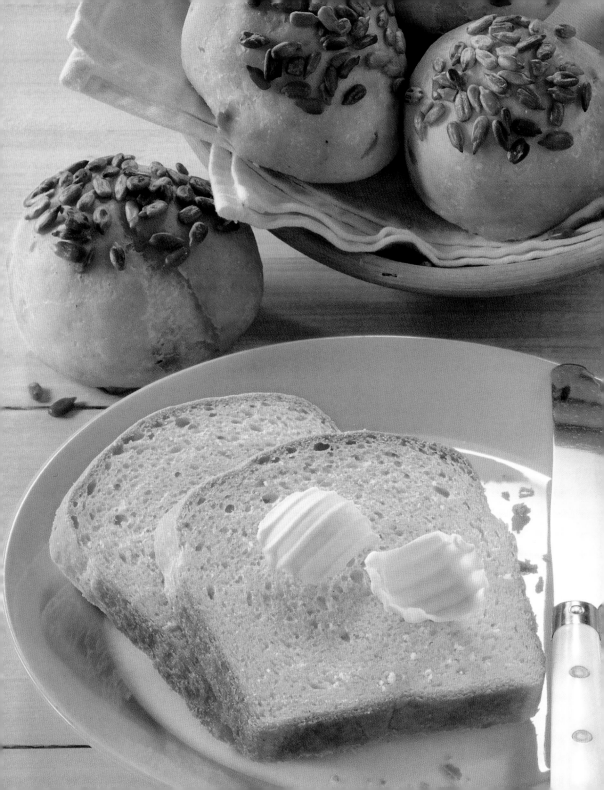

Potato Bread

MAKES 20 SLICES
(1 LOAF TIN 28 CM/11 IN LONG)

butter for greasing
1 cube fresh yeast (42 g/1½ oz)
1 tsp sugar
150 g (5 oz) lukewarm buttermilk
   (or water)
200 g (6½ oz) cooked floury potatoes
500 g (1 lb) gluten-free flour
1 tbsp salt
300 ml (10 fl oz/1¼ cups) lukewarm
   water
2 tbsp oil

PREPARATION about 45 mins
RISING about 30-40 mins
BAKING about 1 hr

NUTRITIONAL VALUES PER PORTION:
110 Cal • 1 g protein • 2 g fat • 22 g carbohydrate

1. Crumble the yeast, stir with the sugar into the buttermilk until smooth and leave to swell for about 10 minutes.

2. Lightly grease the loaf tin. Peel the cooked potatoes and push them through a potato ricer. Knead into a thick dough with the flour, salt, yeast and milk mixture and the lukewarm water. Work in the oil. Fill the dough into the tin. Moisten a spatula and smooth the top. Place the tin in a warm oven to rise for 30–40 minutes (see Tips on page 104).

3. Remove the tin from the oven and preheat the oven to 225°C (430°F)/200°C (390°F) fan-forced (middle shelf). Bake the bread for about 1 hour. After baking, turn it out of the tin and leave to cool on a rack.

VARIATION

The potato bread will be grainier and more aromatic if you stir about 50 g (1²⁄₃ oz) sunflower seeds, buckwheat flakes or chopped walnuts into the dough.

Rice Bread

MAKES 16 SLICES
(1 LOAF TIN 24 CM/9½ IN LONG)

1 cube fresh yeast (42 g/1½ oz)
1 tsp raw sugar
400 ml (14 fl oz/1¾ cups) lukewarm
   water
butter for greasing
250 g (8 oz) rice flour
150 g (5 oz) potato starch
100 g (3⅓ oz) rice bran
2 tsp guar gum
1 tsp salt
1 tsp apple cider vinegar
2 tbsp rapeseed oil for brushing

PREPARATION about 30 mins
RISING about 40 mins
BAKING about 1 hr

NUTRITIONAL VALUES PER PORTION:
125 Cal • 2 g protein • 2 g fat • 26 g carbohydrate

1. Stir together the yeast, sugar and 100 ml (3 fl oz/½ cup) lukewarm water. Leave to rise until bubbles form. Lightly grease the baking tin.

2. Combine the rice flour with the potato starch, rice bran, guar gum and salt. Add the yeast and water mixture, the vinegar and the remaining lukewarm water. Knead everything, ideally using the dough hook of a food processor.

3. Fill the dough into the tin, moisten a spatula and smooth the top. Leave to rise in a warm oven for 30–40 minutes (see Tips on page 104).

4. Remove the tin from the oven and preheat the oven to 225°C (430°F)/200°C (390°F) fan-forced (middle shelf). Bake the bread for 50 minutes, then brush the loaf with the oil and bake for another 10 minutes to finish. After baking, turn out of the tin and leave to cool completely on a wire rack.

VARIATION

If you like, you can add 50 g (1²⁄₃ oz) linseeds, sunflower seeds or ground nuts to the dough. Just use 50 ml (2 fl oz/¼ cup) more water.

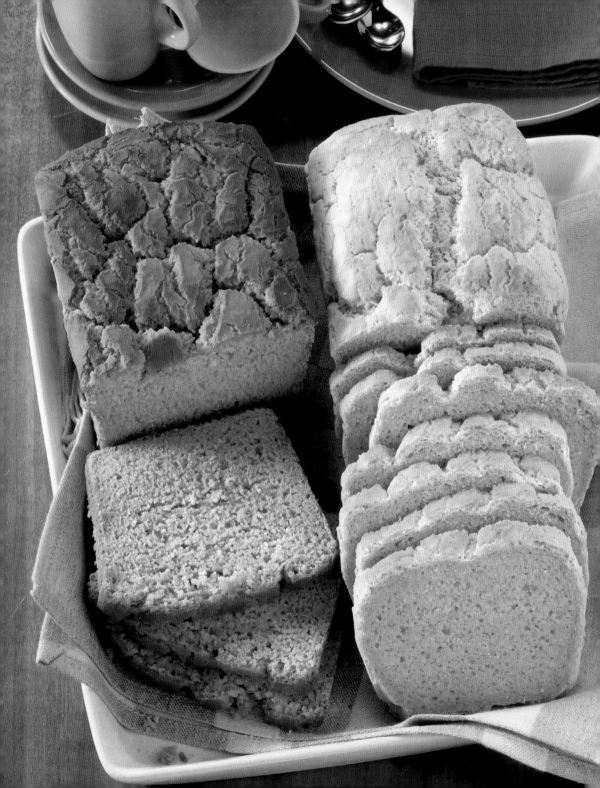

Multigrain Yoghurt Bread

**MAKES 20 SLICES
(1 LONG LOAF)**

400 g (13 oz) gluten-free flour
  mix for country bread

100 g (3⅓ oz) buckwheat flour

1 tsp sugar

1½ tsp dried yeast

2 tsp salt

50 g (1⅔ oz) linseed (flaxseed)

50 g (1⅔ oz) sunflower seeds

200 g (6½ oz) yoghurt

250 ml (8 fl oz/1 cup) lukewarm
  water

4 tbsp rapeseed oil

PREPARATION about 30 mins

RISING about 40 mins

BAKING about 1 hr

1. Combine the two types of flour with the sugar, dried yeast, salt, linseeds and sunflower seeds. Line the baking tray with baking paper.

2. Stir together the yoghurt, the water and 2 tablespoons of the oil. Warm lightly at a low temperature (about 35°C/95°F), then add to the flour mixture. Knead all the ingredients to form a smooth dough – using the dough hook of the food processor.

3. Shape the dough into a longish loaf and place it on the tray. With a sharp knife make a few cuts in the dough, then leave to rise in the warm oven for about 30–40 minutes (see Tips on page 104).

4. Remove the bread from the oven and preheat the oven to 250°C (480°F)/220°C (430°F) fan-forced (middle shelf). Bake the bread for about 10 minutes. Reduce the temperature to 225°C (435°F)/200°C (390°F) fan-forced and bake for a further 40 minutes. Brush the bread with the remaining oil and bake for another 10 minutes to finish. After baking, turn out of the tin and leave on a rack to cool.

TIP

To ensure this bread is also good for lactose intolerance, use a lactose-free yoghurt.

VARIATION

Replace the buckwheat flour with chestnut flour for an extra-hearty country loaf.

NUTRITIONAL VALUES PER PORTION:
130 Cal • 3 g protein • 4 g fat • 21 g carbohydrate

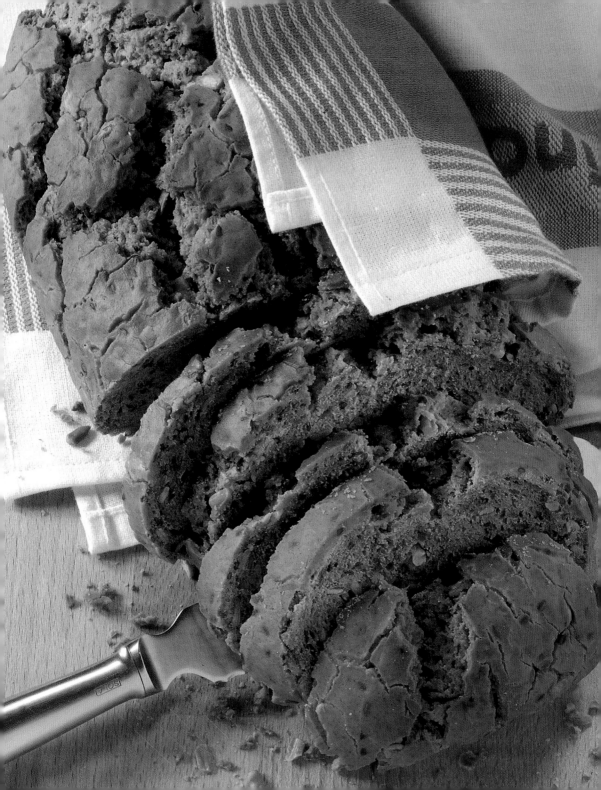

Amaranth Bread with linseed

MAKES 22 SLICES
(1 LOAF TIN 30 CM/12 IN LONG)

butter for greasing

1 cube fresh yeast (42 g/1½ oz)

1 tsp sugar

550 ml (18 fl oz/2⅓ cups) lukewarm
   water

500 g (1 lb) gluten-free plain flour

150 g (5 oz) ground amaranth
   (or buckwheat flour)

1 tsp salt

100 g (3⅓ oz) linseed

1 tbsp apple cider vinegar

2 tbsp rapeseed oil

PREPARATION about 30 mins

RISING about 40 mins

BAKING about 1 hr

1. Crumble the yeast and stir together with the sugar and about 100 ml (3 fl oz/½ cup) water until smooth. Leave to rise for a few minutes until bubbles form. Lightly grease the tin.

2. Knead the flour with the amaranth, salt, linseed, cider vinegar, yeast and water mixture to form a firm dough. Place the dough in the tin, moisten a spatula and smooth the top. Leave to rise in a warm oven for about 30–40 minutes (see Tips on page 104).

3. Remove the tin from the oven and preheat the oven to 250°C (480°F)/220°C (430°F) fan-forced (middle shelf). Bake the bread for 10 minutes, then reduce the temperature to 225°C (435°F)/200°C (390°F) and bake for another 40 minutes. Brush with the oil and bake for another 10 minutes to finish. After baking, turn onto a rack to cool.

TIP

The bread tastes best when freshly baked but it is also suitable for freezing. Cut into slices and freeze, then re-heat as many slices as needed in the toaster.

NUTRITIONAL VALUES PER PORTION:

135 Cal • 3 g protein • 3 g fat • 23 g carbohydrate

Walnut Bread

MAKES 20 SLICES
(1 LOAF TIN 28 CM/11 IN LONG)

butter for greasing

1 cube fresh yeast (42 g/1½ oz)

1 tsp sugar

500 ml (16 fl oz/2 cups)
   lukewarm water

500 g (1 lb) gluten-free bread
   mix (e.g. Casalare)

50 g (1⅔ oz) freshly kibbled linseed
   (flaxseed)

100 g (3⅓ oz) ground amaranth
   (or buckwheat flour)

2 tsp salt

5 tbsp sunflowerseed oil

100 g (3⅓ oz) walnut kernels

PREPARATION about 35 mins

RISING about 40 mins

BAKING about 1 hr

1. Crumble the yeast and stir together with the sugar into 100 ml (3 fl oz/½ cup) lukewarm water until smooth. Leave for a few minutes until bubbles form.

2. Grease the tin. Combine the flour, linseed, amaranth and salt. Add the yeast water mixture, the remaining lukewarm water and 3 tablespoons oil. Knead all the ingredients together, using the dough hook of the food processor. Chop the walnuts and knead into the dough.

3. Fill the dough into the tin. Moisten the spatula and smooth the top. Leave to rise in the warm oven for 30–40 minutes (see Tips on page 104).

4. Remove the tin from the oven and preheat the oven to 250°C (480°F)/220°C (430°F) fan-forced (middle shelf). Bake for 10 minutes initially, then reduce the temperature to 225°C (435°F)/200°C (390°F) fan-forced and continue baking for another 40 minutes. Brush the bread with 2 tablespoons oil and bake for another 10 minutes to finish. After baking, turn out and leave to cool on a rack.

NUTRITIONAL VALUES PER PORTION:

170 Cal • 3 g protein • 7 g fat • 25 g carbohydrate

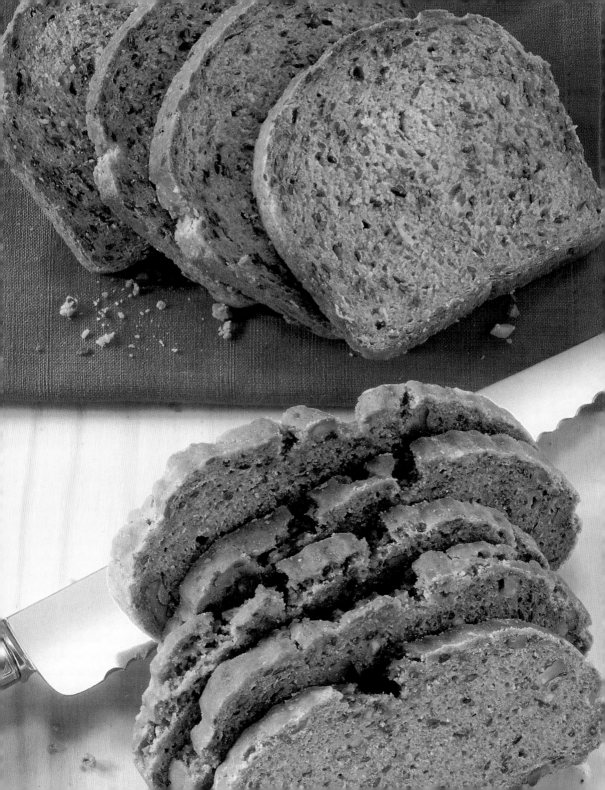

Bread without using a bread mix

**MAKES 16 SLICES
(1 BREAD TIN
24 CM/9½ IN LONG)**

1½ tsp dried yeast

1 tsp sugar

400 ml (14 fl oz/1¾ cups) lukewarm
   water

butter for greasing

200 g (6½ oz) rice flour

150 g (5 oz) cornflour (cornstarch)

150 g (5 oz) buckwheat flour

2 tsp xanthan gum or guar gum
   (thickener)

1½ tsp salt

1 tsp apple cider vinegar

2 tbsp rapeseed oil for brushing

PREPARATION about 30 mins

RISING about 30-40 mins

BAKING about 1 hr

1. Stir the yeast with the sugar into 100 ml (3 fl oz/½ cup) lukewarm water until smooth. Leave to rise for a few minutes until bubbles form. Lightly grease the baking tin.

2. Combine the rice flour with the cornflour, buckwheat flour, guar gum and salt. Add the yeast water, vinegar and the rest of the 300 ml (10 fl oz/1¼ cups) lukewarm water and knead thoroughly for at least 3 minutes – if possible, using the dough hook of a food processor.

3. Fill the dough into the tin, moisten a spatula and smooth the top. Leave the bread to rise for 30–40 minutes in a warm oven (see Tips on page 104). The dough should rise in volume by about one-third.

4. Remove the tin from the oven and preheat the oven to 250°C (480°F)/220°C (430°F) fan-forced (middle shelf). Bake the bread for 10 minutes, then reduce the temperature to 225°C (435°F)/200°C (390°F) fan-forced and bake for another 40 minutes. Brush the bread with oil and bake for another 10 minutes to finish. Turn out of the tin and leave to cool on a rack.

TIPS

You can create your own combination of different flours, using cornflour, buckwheat, amaranth, chestnut, quinoa, millet, tapioca or other flours. The quantity should come to 500 g (1 lb) in total, and you should also include a thickener for example xanthan gum.

The cider vinegar helps the dough rise. Instead of water you can also use sparkling mineral water, buttermilk or yoghurt.

Add 30 g (1 oz) nuts, sunflower seeds or linseeds to give the bread a different flavour.

NUTRITIONAL VALUES PER PORTION:
130 Cal • 2 g protein • 2 g fat • 26 g carbohydrate

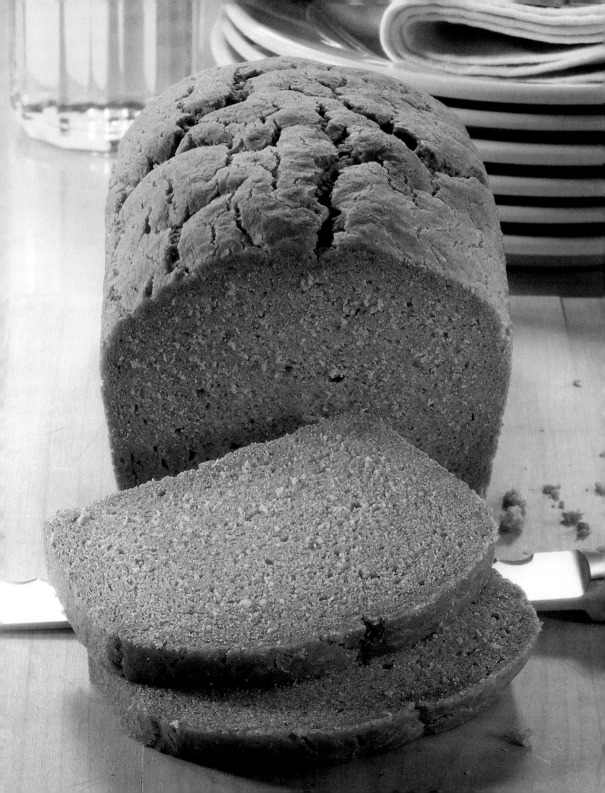

My Favourite Bread

**MAKES 22 SLICES
(1 ROUND LOAF TIN
30 CM/12 IN DIAMETER)**

1 cube fresh yeast (42 g/1½ oz)

1 tsp sugar

530 ml (17 fl oz/2⅓ cups) lukewarm
water

butter for greasing

500 g (1 lb) gluten-free
plain flour

50 g (1⅔ oz) buckwheat flour

50 g (1⅔ oz) linseed (flaxseed)

50 g (1⅔ oz) millet flakes

50 g (1⅔ oz) soy flakes

50 g (1⅔ oz) sunflower seeds

2 tsp salt

1 tbsp apple cider vinegar

3 tbsp rapeseed oil

gluten-free breadcrumbs
for sprinkling

PREPARATION about 30 mins

RISING about 40 mins

BAKING about 1 hr

1. Crumble the yeast and stir together with the sugar and 100 ml (3 fl oz/½ cup) lukewarm water until smooth. Leave to swell for a few minutes until bubbles form. Grease the baking tin and sprinkle with gluten-free breadcrumbs.

2. Combine the flour with the buckwheat flour, linseed, millet flakes, soy flakes, sunflower seeds and salt. Add the yeast water, vinegar, 1 tablespoon oil and the remaining water and thoroughly knead everything for about 5 minutes – ideally using the dough hook of a food processor.

3. Place the dough into a loaf tin. Moisten a spatula and smooth the top. Leave to rise in a warm oven for about 30–40 minutes (see Tips on page 104). The dough should increase in volume by about half.

4. Remove the tin from the oven then preheat th oven to 225°C (435°F)/200°C (390°F) fan-forced (middle shelf). Bake the bread for 50 minutes, then brush it with 2 tablespoons oil and bake for another 10 minutes to finish. After baking, turn out and leave to cool on a rack.

TIP

If you want to bake this bread in a breadmaker, use 650 ml (21 fl oz/2¾ cups) water.

VARIATION

Why not bake a delicious walnut bread for a change? Instead of the 530 ml (17 fl oz/2⅓ cups) water use half and half lukewarm water and lukewarm buttermilk, plus substitute 50 g (1⅔ oz) chopped walnuts for the sunflower seeds.

NUTRITIONAL VALUES PER PORTION:
145 Cal • 3 g protein • 4 g fat • 23 g carbohydrate

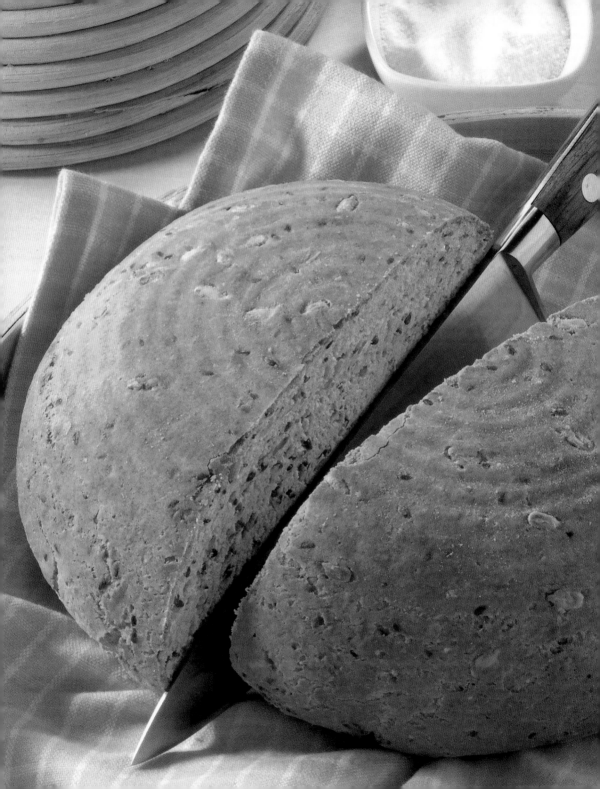

GLOSSARY

BAKING TIPS

> Gluten-free baking works best when the ingredients are at room temperature.
> Gluten-free bread dough should be baked as soon as it has been proofed once, as it often turns out poorly the second time around.
> Gluten-free dough needs to be very moist in order to rise. The following method has been tried and tested: briefly heat the oven to 50°C (120°F), then switch off (about 35°C/95°F). Place the dough on a tray or in a pan or bowl, and put in the oven. Slide a rack on top, and cover with a damp tea towel. Make sure the tea towel is removed before baking!
> Moisture is also very important in the actual baking process, as it prevents the bread from drying out. During baking, you should therefore fill an ovenproof container with water and place this in the oven, even if you use a convection oven.
> The gluten-free dough may have a different consistency to normal bread dough before baking. Wrapping the dough in cling film allows it to form a loaf more easily.
> Gluten-free bread can be made more moist by adding strained, boiled potatoes.

BINDING AGENTS

Gluten is partly responsible for the favourable baking properties of plain flour. It binds the dough and makes the bread elastic. If there is no gluten, this property thus sometimes has to be substituted by other binding agents. Guar, carob or arrowroot starch are good options.

Use around 2 tsp for one bread loaf.

BINDING SAUCES

Soups and sauces often have to be thickened slightly, and there are various ways of doing this, for example with starch, rice flour or gluten-free flour. Simply mix with water and stir into the soup or sauce.

CLEANLINESS

When preparing gluten-free food, make sure everything in the kitchen is spotlessly clean, because even small amounts of gluten can trigger symptoms. Baking pans must be cleaned thoroughly; separate pans should ideally be used for gluten-free baking. Silicone bakeware is excellent for cooking gluten-free food. If trays and pans are also used for normal baking, these can be laid with baking paper if necessary. The gluten-free ingredients should also be stored in sealed containers to prevent any gluten contamination.

DESSERTS

Make sure ice creams and other purchased desserts are gluten-free. The food and ingredients lists published by the Coeliac Society of Australia are very helpful in determining whether a dessert can be enjoyed freely or will cause more pain than pleasure.

EATING AT RESTAURANTS

There is no problem eating gluten-free meals at most restaurants. Simply speak to the waiters and explain what you can and can't eat. The Coeliac Society provides a Restaurant Card to help communicate what foods are safe for you to have. You can pass this onto the chef in the kitchen. The card is available in more than 35 different languages, which is particularly helpful when you are travelling overseas or dining at foreign restaurants.

EATING ON PLANES

When travelling by air, you should make it clear when booking your flights that you require gluten-free meals; the airlines can usually cater for this. Double-check this again the day before departure and at check-in to make sure all is in order. However, it is still advisable to have some gluten-free bread or crackers in your hand luggage, in case the flight attendants are not totally familiar with the issue and end up serving you normal bread.

HIDDEN GLUTEN

Make sure baking ingredients such as baking powder, chocolate icing, spices, flavouring, marzipan or similar are definitely gluten-free, as they sometimes contain hidden ingredients like malt, wheat starch and so on. The Coeliac Society of Australia's ingredients list tells you which products you can use.

ITALIAN PIZZA

Just because you have coeliac disease, doesn't mean you can't have Italian-style pizza. Some places are now offering gluten-free pizzas. Alternatively bring your own gluten-free pizza base with you, and add the topping you want. A quick call in advance is usually all that is needed to ensure the kitchen is informed and okay with your special request. Once at the restaurant, make sure the waiter is aware that the pizza must be baked on a thoroughly cleaned tray, and not on the floury oven slab, to prevent it from coming into contact with glutenous flour.

LACTOSE-FREE

If you have a lactose intolerance, you can substitute butter with lactose-free margarines in the recipes. Supermarkets sell lactose-free yoghurt, milk, cream and curd cheese. The fermentation of hard cheese means it contains very little lactose. In these cases, you must find out exactly how much lactose you can tolerate.

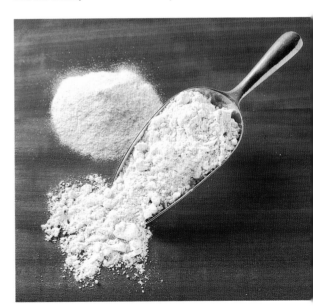

MIXING FLOUR YOURSELF

Gluten-free flour mixes are very helpful and often have very similar baking properties to normal wheat flour. If you want to mix your own flour, here are a few suggestions:

> 200 g (6½ oz) cornflour, 150 g (5 oz) rice flour, 150 g (5 oz) potato starch
> 200 g (6½ oz) buckwheat flour, 150 g (5 oz) cornflour, 150 g (5 oz) tapioca flour
> 200 g (6½ oz) rice flour, 150 g (5 oz) amaranth (ground), 150 g (5 oz) potato starch

Try out your own combinations and find the one you like best. Add 2 teaspoons binding agent, for example psyllium, carob gum, guar gum or arrowroot to each of the flour mixtures.

OPTIONS FOR PURCHASING GLUTEN-FREE FOOD

Health food shops contain a wide variety of gluten-free foods, and some online stores also sell gluten-free products.

If you shop for gluten-free products at a supermarket, you should always consult the ingredient list published by The Coeliac Society of Australia to be sure of what you buy.

There are also a number of gluten-free foods available to buy online. Try, for example:

>www.glutenfreeforme.com.au
>www.glutenfreeeatingdirectory.com.au
>www.glutenfreeshop.com.au
>www.myglutenfreesupermarketguide.com.au

PSYLLIUM (FIBRE HUSK)

So-called psyllium (psyllium plantago) is an ideal binding agent used to improve the processing and baking properties of bread. It swells easily, enabling it to absorb a lot of fluid which is retained in gluten-free baking. Psyllium is the seed husk of a plantain species. It has only recently started to be incorporated into gluten-free cooking, but is once again being used as a component in some ready-mixed flours due to its favourable properties.

Stir 1–2 tsp into the liquid required for the bread (lukewarm water or buttermilk, for example), leave to swell for about 10 minutes, then add the mixture to the dough. Proceed as usual. Ground psyllium is sold as psyllium (fibre) husk powder under brands such as The Gluten Free Company (see manufacturer's list on page 123), but you can also buy it whole from pharmacies and grind it yourself.

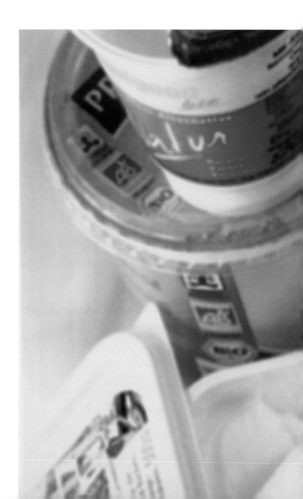

SIDE DISHES

Recommended side dishes to cook at home or choose in a restaurant include rice, potatoes or gluten-free noodles (see manufacturer's list on page 123).

STORAGE

Gluten-free bread tastes delicious if it is frozen in slices, and the frozen slices are then crisped up in the toaster as and when they are needed. You must, however, keep a separate toaster for the gluten-free toasts. Also, make absolutely sure you always store the gluten-free bread away from bread containing gluten – keep it in its own bag or bread tin.

USING OLD RECIPES

You can still keep using most of your favourite recipes although these may contain gluten. The flour used can generally be substituted by an appropriate gluten-free flour (see the manufacturer's list on page 123), though this may alter the baking properties somewhat, that is, gluten-free flour generally needs more liquid. Adding binding agents helps ensure the processing and baking properties are as similar as possible to those of glutenous flour.

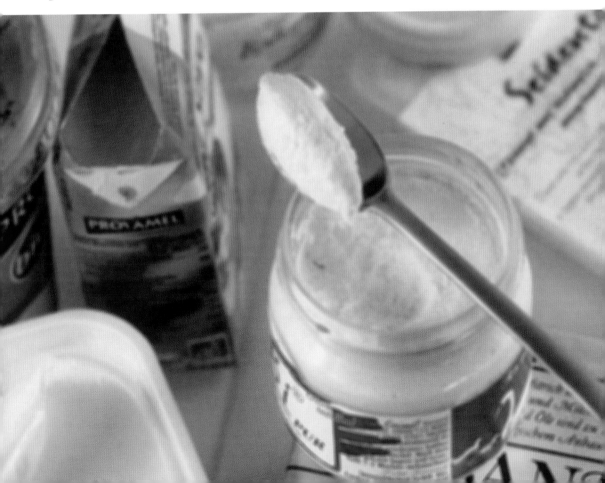

What your first weekly menu plan might look like	Breakfast	Snack
DAY 1	Millet muesli with apples	Carrot and cucumber
DAY 2	Yeast-free bread roll with jam (p. 106)	Natural yoghurt with berries
DAY 3	Natural yoghurt with dried fruits and nuts	Apple turnovers (p. 58 Var.)
DAY 4	Walnut bread with hard cheese (p. 114)	Carrot and celery
DAY 5	Natural yoghurt with fresh fruits	Carrot and cucumber
DAY 6	My favourite bread with ham (p. 118)	Buttermilk with raspberries
DAY 7	Weekend bread roll with jam (p. 104)	Honeydew melon

Delicious meals free from gluten – the first week at a glance

EXTRA TIP: Of course you don't have to bake fresh bread or rolls every single day. Both bread in slices and individual rolls can easily be frozen and then thawed as and when you need them. You can pop bread slices still frozen straight into the toaster, or place rolls in a cafe-style sandwich press. Bake cakes and pastries whenever you feel like it.

Lunch	Snack	Supper
Lasagne (p. 36)	Coconut and orange muffins (p. 78)	Walnut bread with turkey breast fillet (p. 114)
Burritos with chicken filling (p. 44)	Nut croissants (p. 58 Var.)	Cream of mushroom soup (p. 26)
Penne with zucchini sauce (p. 34)	Grapes	Potato bread with herb cream cheese and tomatoes (p. 110)
Leek quiche (p. 60)	Apple cake with cinnamon frosting (p. 90)	Prosciutto croissants (p. 58 Var.)
Gnocchi (p. 30) with tasty tomato sauce (p. 28)	Chocolate and almond muffins (p. 76)	French onion tart (p. 54)
Polenta pizza (p. 52)	Raspberry tiramisu (p. 72)	Focaccia (p. 48)
Pickled beef roast with bread dumplings (p. 40) Sweet millet gratin (p. 70)	Linzer Torte (p. 92)	Pancake wraps with meat filling (p. 42)

Food item	Not permitted
CEREAL	wheat, rye, oat, barley, unripe spelt grains, spelt, wheat, triticale
CEREAL PRODUCTS	baked goods and cereal products such as semolina, pearl barley, flakes, coarse meal, bran, pasta and sprouts of the aforementioned cereals, breadcrumbs, croutons, muesli, ready-made mixes, popcorn and cornflakes
VEGETABLES	frozen vegetables and tinned vegetables with vague composition
TUBERS AND PULSES	potato products such as ready-made potato batter, ready-made potato dumplings, croquettes, purée, salad, chips and French fries
READY-MADE MEALS, FROZEN FOODS, TINNED FOOD	ready-made meals and commercially-produced foodstuffs, sauces, soups, desserts, sweets and potato products with unclear ingredients
NUTS AND SEEDS	
FRUIT	fruit preparations and fruit fillings with additives, thickened fruits, dried fruit (possibly containing sulphur), fruit bars
EGGS	
MILK AND DAIRY PRODUCTS	milk products with additives, fruit preparations or cereals, milk-based drinks, reduced fat products, cheese preparations, processed cheese, blue cheese, cheese with cereal-based rind, light cheese, herb butter
MEAT AND MEAT PRODUCTS	meat products such as cold cuts, pâté and sausages, meat preparations such as hamburgers, meat fillings, breaded meat, meat in sauces with unclear ingredients meat pies
SEAFOOD	fish products and tinned fish with unclear ingredients, breaded fish, fish fingers, deep-fried fish, surimi
FATS AND OILS	oils, margarine and butter, mayonnaise, reduced fat products, light products with additives that might contain gluten
SPREADS	nut and nougat spreads, spreads with ingredients that might contain gluten
DRINKS	based drinks, coffee and cocoa from vending machines, flavoured teas, beer and other malt-based drinks, lemonade, sherberts, coke, fruit juice drinks containing dietary fibre, juices with additives, liqueurs, whiskeys, brandies, rum, gin, whiskey, schnapps
CONFECTIONARY AND SNACKS	snack products based on potatoes or maize, candied products, coated products, all confectionary, chocolate, pralines, marzipan, liquorice, ice cream, jelly babies, candies, creams, custards, desserts, sweet chilled soups, coatings, fruit bars with additives that might contain gluten
"LIGHT" PRODUCTS	all light products with unclear ingredients
INGREDIENTS	additives, flavourings, preservatives, flavour enhancers, various thickeners, baking powder, cake glazes, spice mixtures, seasoning blends, seasoning mixes, vegetable stock
VARIOUS	seitan, fried onions, salad dressings, mustard, soy sauce, tomato sauce, tomato concentrate with ingredients that might contain gluten

If in doubt check the Ingredient List from Coeliac Australia! Take extra care with medications, dental care and oral hygiene products, dental prostheses products, lipsticks and lipcare products!

Restricted, or only gluten-free diet products	Permitted
	rice, wild rice, corn, millet, buckwheat, quinoa, amaranth
special products such as gluten-free breads, baked goods, pasta, baking mixes	baked goods, cereal products, pasta and sprouts made from the permitted cereals listed above
tinned vegetables without additives	all fresh vegetables and herbs, pure frozen vegetables
in potato products only those that are gluten-free or gluten-free diet products	potatoes and potato starch, sweet potatoes, tapioca, beans, peas, lentils, soy beans
gluten-free products and those products especially developed for a gluten-free diet containing the label "gluten-free"	
	all nuts, chestnuts, sunflower seeds, pumpkin seeds, sesame seeds, poppy seeds, linseed, coconut
in preparations only gluten-free products or gluten-free diet products	all fresh fruits, unsulphurised dried fruits
egg dishes only if containing permitted cereals or gluten-free or gluten-free diet products	all types of eggs
all dairy products without additives or ingredients that may contain gluten; in preparations only gluten-free or gluten-free diet products	pure milk products, whey, as long as no lactose intolerance has been diagnosed
gluten-free meat preparations	all kinds of meat, poultry and game
fish products and tinned fish without additives that may contain gluten	fresh and smoked fish, crustaceans
margarine, mayonnaise without additives that may contain gluten	all pure oils, butter, lard, pure fat, peanut butter, pure mayonnaise
spreads without ingredients or additives that may contain gluten	honey, jam/marmalade, sugar beet molasses, almond paste, nut purée, tahini
instant coffee, cereal coffee, malt coffee, ready-made coffee drinks, cocoa, milk-drinks that are gluten-free according to the Ingredient List from Coeliac Australia	pure teas without additives, pure juices, freshly brewed coffee, mineral water, soy drinks, wine, champagne
gluten-free products and products specially produced for a gluten-free diet	sugar, caramel
gluten-free products and products specially produced for a gluten-free diet	
gluten-free products and products specially produced for a gluten-free diet	guar gum, locust bean gum (carob bean gum), kuzu, pectin, arrowroot, carageen, vinegar without spice mixes or malt, all pure spices and mixtures of these, lecithin
products without glutenous additives	tofu, algae

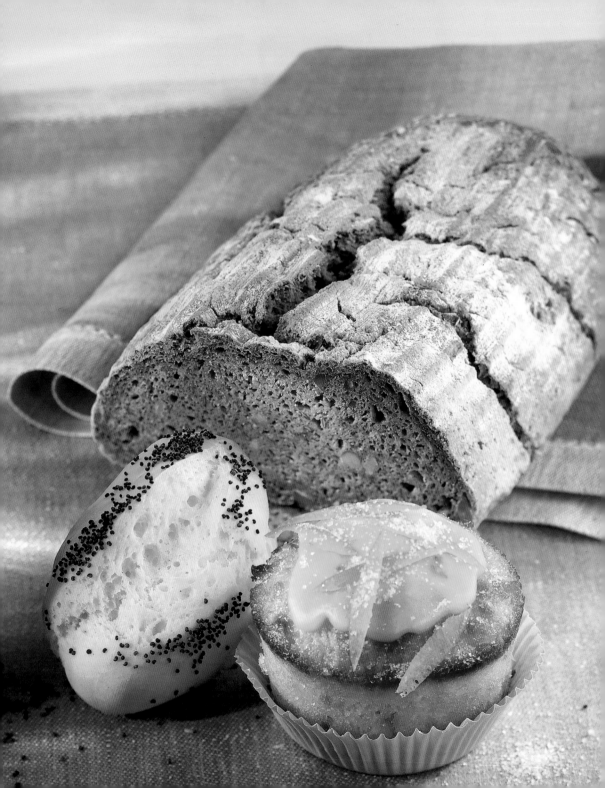

RECIPES INDEX – BY CHAPTER

SOUPS AND SAUCES

béchamel sauce 28
cream of mushroom soup 26
creamy curry sauce 29
spicy barbecue sauce 29
tasty tomato sauce 28
vegetable soup with polenta gnocci 26

PASTA DISHES

cheesy polenta bake 32
gnocchi with parmesan 30
lasagne 36
meaty pasta parcels 38
penne with zucchini sauce 34
spaghetti carbonara 34

MAIN COURSES

burritos with chicken filling 44
pancake wraps with meat filling 42
pickled beef roast with bread dumplings 40
zucchini tortilla 46

SAVOURY BAKING

basic recipe cream cheese and oil pastry 56
basic recipe cream cheese puff pastry 56
basic recipe pizza dough 48
basic recipe yeast dough 54
cheese bites 62
colourful family pizza 50
focaccia 48
French onion tart 54
leek quiche 60
meat parcels 58
polenta pizza 52

DESSERTS

basic recipe sponge cake 72
Belgian waffles 68
French apple crumble 64
German cream cheese potato cakes 68
light orange mousse 66
raspberry tiramisu 72
red jelly with custard 64
rice and cream cheese gratin with apples 70
Scandinavian buttermilk cream 66
sweet millet gratin 70

CAKES AND GATEAUX

almond cake 86
almond slice 78
apple cake with cinnamon frosting 90
basic recipe shortcrust pastry 88
buckwheat cake 80
cheesecake without base 74
chocolate and almond muffins 76
coconut & orange muffins 78
espresso cake 80
French cherry gâteau 82
fruity walnut muffins 76
gooseberry cake 90
lemon cake 82
Linzer torte 92
raspberry cream cake 74
rhubarb cake with custard topping 88
Swiss carrot cake 84

CHRISTMAS BAKING

almond crescents 100
butter biscuits 94
chocolate slices 100
coconut & marzipan macaroons 98
fancy pistachio fingers 96
hazelnut macaroons 98
lemon hearts 96
mini meringues 102
walnut cookies 102

BREADS AND ROLLS

amaranth bread with linseed 114
bread without using a bread mix 116
yeast-free bread rolls 106
multigrain yoghurt bread 112
my favourite bread 118
potato bread 110
rice bread 110
walnut bread 114
weekend bread rolls 104
white bread rolls or white bread 108
wholemeal bread rolls or wholemeal bread 106

INDEX

Almonds
almond cake 86
almond slice 78
almond crescents 100
apple cake with cinnamon frosting 90
basic recipe sponge cake (variation) 72
Belgian waffles (variation) 68
buckwheat cake 80
butter biscuits 94
cheese bites 62
chocolate and almond muffins 76
chocolate slices 100
fancy pistachio fingers 96
French apple crumble 64
gooseberry cake 90
hazelnut cookies (variation) 98
lemon hearts 96
Linzer torte 92
meat parcels (sweet variation) 58
mini meringues 102
raspberry cream cake 74
raspberry tiramisu 72
rice and cream cheese gratin with apples 70
Scandinavian buttermilk cream 66
sweet millet gratin (variation) 70
Swiss carrot cake 84
walnut cookies 102
almond cake 86
almond slice 78
almond crescents 100
amaranth bread with linseed 114
Apples
apple cake with cinnamon frosting 90
French apple crumble 64

meat parcels (sweet variation) 58
rice and cream cheese gratin with apples 70
sweet millet gratin (variation) 70
apple cake with cinnamon frosting 90

barbecue sauce, spicy 29
basic recipe cream cheese puff pastry 56
basic recipe cream cheese and oil pastry 56
basic recipe pizza dough 48
basic recipe shortcrust pastry 88
basic recipe sponge cake 72
basic recipe yeast dough 54
béchamel sauce 28
Belgian waffles 68
bread without using a bread mix 116
buckwheat cake 80
burritos with chicken filling 44
butter biscuits 94

cheese bites 62
cheesecake without base 74
cheesy polenta bake 32
Cherries
cheesecake without base (variation) 74
French cherry gâteau 82
fruity walnut muffins 76
red jelly with custard 64
Scandinavian buttermilk cream (variation) 66
cherry gâteau, French 82
chocolate slices 100
chocolate and almond muffins 76
cinnamon frosting, apple cake with 90
coconut & marzipan macaroons 98

coconut & orange muffins 78
colourful family pizza 50
Cream Cheese
basic recipe cream cheese and oil pastry 56
basic recipe cream cheese puff pastry 56
basic recipe yeast dough 54
cheese bites 62
cheesecake without base 74
German cream cheese potato cakes 68
gnocchi with parmesan 30
meat parcels 58
raspberry cream cake 74
raspberry tiramisu 72
rice and cream cheese gratin with apples 70
yeast-free bread rolls 106
cream cheese puff pastry, basic recipe 56
cream cheese and oil pastry, basic recipe 56
cream of mushroom soup 26
creamy curry sauce 29
custard, red jelly with 64

espresso cake 80

family pizza, colourful 50
fancy pistachio fingers 96
favourite bread, my 118
focaccia 48
French apple crumble 64
French cherry gâteau 82
French onion tart 54
fruity walnut muffins 76

German cream cheese potato cakes 68

gnocchi with parmesan 30

gooseberry cake 90

Hazelnuts
apple cake with cinnamon frosting 90
buckwheat cake (variation) 80
espresso cake 80
French cherry gâteau 82
hazelnut macaroons 98
meat parcels (sweet variation) 58
sweet millet gratin 70
Swiss carrot cake 84

hazelnut macaroons 98

lasagne 36

leek quiche 60

lemon hearts 96

lemon cake 82

light orange mousse 66

Linzer torte 92

Marzipan
almond crescents 100
chocolate and almond muffins (variation) 76
coconut & marzipan macaroons 98
coconut & orange muffins 78
Swiss carrot cake 84

meat parcels 58

meaty pasta parcels 38

millet gratin, sweet 70

mini meringues 102

Muffins
fruity walnut muffins 76
chocolate and almond muffins 76
coconut & orange muffins 78

multigrain yoghurt bread 112

my favourite bread 118

orange mousse, light 66

pancake wraps with meat filling 42

penne with zucchini sauce 34

pickled beef roast with bread dumplings 40

pistachio fingers, fancy 96

pizza dough, basic recipe 48

polenta pizza 52

potato bread 110

Raspberries
fruity walnut muffins (variation) 76
raspberry cream cake 74
raspberry tiramisu 72
red jelly with custard 64

raspberry cream cake 74

raspberry tiramisu 72

red jelly with custard 64

rhubarb cake with custard topping 88

rice bread 110

rice and cream cheese gratin with apples 70

Scandinavian buttermilk cream 66

Shortcrust Pastry
apple cake with cinnamon frosting 90
basic recipe shortcrust pastry 88
gooseberry cake 90
rhubarb cake with custard topping 88

spaghetti carbonara 34

spicy barbecue sauce 29

Strawberries
Belgian waffles (Tip) 68
fruity walnut muffins (variation) 76
red jelly with custard 64
Scandinavian buttermilk cream 66

sweet millet gratin 70

Swiss carrot cake 84

tomato sauce, tasty 28

vegetable soup with polenta gnocchi 26

waffles, Belgian 68

Walnuts
fruity walnut muffins 76
hazelnut macaroons (variation) 98
my favourite bread (variation) 118
potato bread (variation) 110
walnut bread 114
walnut cookies 102

walnut bread 114

walnut cookies 102

walnut muffins, fruity 76

weekend bread rolls 104

white bread rolls or white bread 108

wholemeal bread rolls or wholemeal bread 106

Yeast Dough
amaranth bread w. linseed 114
basic recipe pizza dough 48
basic recipe yeast dough 54
bread without using a bread mix 116
colourful family pizza 50
focaccia 48
French onion tart 54
multigrain yoghurt bread 112
my favourite bread 118
potato bread 110
rice bread 110
walnut bread 114
weekend bread rolls 104
white bread rolls or white bread 108
wholemeal bread rolls or wholemeal bread 106

yeast-free bread rolls 106

yoghurt bread, multigrain 112

zucchini tortilla 46

This edition published in 2015 by New Holland Publishers Pty Ltd
London • Sydney • Auckland

Unit 9, The Chandlery, 50 Westminster Bridge Road, London SE1 7QY, United Kingdom
1/66 Gibbes Street, Chatswood, NSW 2067, Australia
218 Lake Road, Northcote, Auckland 0627, New Zealand

www.newhollandpublishers.com

Published originally under the title Gluten-Free Cooking by Trudel Marquardt and Britta-Marei Lanzenberger
ISBN 3-7742-8797, © 2005 Gräfe und Unzer Verlag GmbH, München

A record of this book is held at the British Library and the National Library of Australia.
ISBN 9781742576329

DISCLAIMER: The nutritional information for each recipe is an estimate only and may vary depending on the brand of
ingredients used and due to natural biological variations in the composition of natural foods such as meat, fish, fruit and
vegetables. All information provided in this book is intended to be a guide only, it does not replace medical advice. Any
concerns readers have about their diet should be discussed with their doctor. Whilst all reasonable efforts have been made
to ensure the accuracy of the information, the Publisher accepts no responsibility for the accuracy of that information or
for any error or omission and shall not be responsible for any decisions made based on such information.

Managing Director: Fiona Schultz
Publisher: Alan Whiticker
Project Editor: Angela Sutherland
Designer: Thomas Casey
Production Director: Olga Dementiev
Printer: Toppan Leefung Printing Ltd

10 9 8 7 6 5 4 3 2 1

Keep up with New Holland Publishers on Facebook
www.facebook.com/NewHollandPublishers